649
Mo

$9.95

Moloney, Kathleen
  Parents' guide to
feeding your kids
right

DATE DUE

SE 8'90			
SE 22'90			
FE 6'92			
FE 21'92			
03			
FEB 01 95			
11/2/96			
MAY 20 97			
MY 17 00			
FE 24 05			
FE 13 09			

DEMCO

Also in the Children's Television Workshop Family
Living Series

*Parents' Guide to Raising Kids Who Love to Learn:
Infant to Grade School*

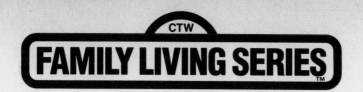

Parents' Guide to

Feeding Your Kids Right

Birth Through Teen Years

• • • • • • • • • • • • • •

CHILDREN'S TELEVISION WORKSHOP

Written by Kathleen Moloney

Preface by Jane Brody

Prentice Hall Press

• • • • • • • • • • • • • •

New York   London   Toronto   Sydney   Tokyo

CHILDREN'S TELEVISION WORKSHOP:

Chairman—Chief Executive Officer: Joan Ganz Cooney
President: David Britt
Publisher: Nina Link

Series Editor: Marge Kennedy
Associate Editor: Sima Bernstein
Nutrition Consultant: Kathleen Carpenter, M.S., R.D.

 Prentice Hall Press
Gulf+Western Building
One Gulf+Western Plaza
New York, New York 10023

Library of Congress Cataloging-in-Publication Data
Moloney, Kathleen.
    Parents' guide to feeding your kids right: birth through teen/
    by Children's Television Workshop: preface by Jane Brody.—1st
    ed.
        p.   cm.—(Children's Television Workshop family living
    series)
    Bibliography: p.
    Includes index.
    ISBN 0-13-649914-7 (pbk.): $9.95.
    1. Children—Nutrition.   I. Children's Television Workshop.
    II. Title. III. Series.
    RJ206.M75 1989
    649'.3—dc19

Designed by Laurence Alexander and Patricia Fabricant

Manufactured in the United States of America

10 9 8 7 6 5 4 3 2 1

First Edition

Acknowledgments

• • • • • •

The editors wish to thank PJ Dempsey of Prentice Hall Press for the knowledge and assistance she offered in preparing and editing this series. We also wish to acknowledge the many contributions of Jane Brody, our preface writer, and our advisory panel, whose names and affiliations are listed on pages vii–ix; the writer of this volume, Kathleen Moloney; and researchers Diane O'Connell, Jeanette Leardi, and Judith Rovenger.

Advisory Panel

• • • • • •

JANE BRODY, our preface writer, is the *New York Times* personal-health columnist. Her widely read and quoted column is carried by more than 100 newspapers around the country. Ms. Brody has also written scores of magazine articles and writes a regular column, "Nutrition Update," for *Family Circle* magazine. As a noted authority on health and nutrition, she has appeared on hundreds of radio and television shows. She is the author of five books, including *New York Times* bestsellers *Jane Brody's Nutrition Book* and *Jane Brody's Good Food Book*.

KATHLEEN CARPENTER, M.S., R.D., is the Director of the Special Supplemental Food Program for Women, Infants, and Children (WIC) at the Albert Einstein College of Medicine. Her program provides a monthly food supplement and nutrition and health counseling to more than 5,000 low-income women, infants, and children. Ms. Carpenter is a former editor of *Environmental Nutrition Newsletter* and coauthor of the textbook *Nutrition and Health*.

ISOBEL CONTENTO, Ph.D., is Chairperson of the Department of Nutrition Education at Teachers College/Columbia University. She is well known in her field for her research on how children and adolescents choose foods. Dr. Contento has been a consultant for numerous nutrition-education programs, including New York State's "Nutrition Comes Alive" curriculum, The American Cancer Society/National Cancer Institute, and UNESCO, Paris.

LAURENCE FINBERG, M.D., is Professor and Chairman, Department of Pediatrics, SUNY Health Science Center at Brooklyn. Dr. Finberg also chairs the American Academy of Pediatrics Nutrition Committee and serves on the editorial boards of *Pediatric Nutrition and Gastroenterology, Journal of American College of Nutrition,* and *American Journal of Diseases of Children.* Dr. Finberg is a past president of the American Board of Pediatrics.

SAMUEL J. FOMON, M.D., is Professor of Pediatrics in the College of Medicine, University of Iowa, and an expert in nutrition of normal infants. His research in this area has resulted in many publications and several books. He has served as Chairman of the Committee on Nutrition of the American Academy of Pediatrics; Expert in Nutrition to the Bureau of Health Care, Delivery, and Assistance; and President of the American Society for Clinical Nutrition. He is currently President of the American Institute of Nutrition.

JO-ANN HESLIN, M.A., R.D., is a registered dietitian, nutrition consultant, and author. Ms. Heslin has written eight books on nutrition. She serves as Associate Editor for the *Journal of Nutrition for the Elderly* and is a member of the editorial advisory boards of *American Baby* magazine and *Environmental Nutrition Newsletter.* Ms. Heslin also writes a regular column for *Childbirth Educator* magazine and is a member of the continuing-education faculty of the School of Nursing, Adelphi University.

NORGE W. JEROME, Ph.D., is the Director of the Office of Nutrition, Bureau for Science and Technology, for the United States Agency for International Development (AID). Prior to this appointment she was a Professor in the Department of Preventive Medicine, University of Kansas School of Medicine. As a pioneer in nutritional anthropology, Dr. Jerome has conducted extensive studies both in the United States and abroad. She has published widely and serves on numerous national and international committees, councils, and panels concerned with nutrition.

MARGARET MCWILLIAMS, Ph.D., R.D., is Professor of Food and Nutrition and Coordinator of Health-Related Programs at California State University, Los Angeles. She has written extensively on nutrition and has been involved with numerous television and radio projects on food and health. Her publications in children's nutrition include *Parents' Nutrition Book* and *Nutrition for the Growing Years.*

HANNA NUBA, M.S., is Director of The New York Public Library Early Childhood Resource and Information Center. She holds a master's degree from Columbia University as well as certification in education and library science from the University of the State of New York. Her publications include *Resources for Early Childhood* and *Infants: Research and Resources.*

ISTAR SCHWAGER, Ph.D., is Director of Research for the Children's Television Workshop magazines—including the *Sesame Street Magazine/Parents' Guide.* She has worked on the development of television shows, books, toys, and other products. She holds a doctorate in educational psychology and a master's degree in early childhood education. Dr. Schwager has taught at levels from preschool to graduate school and writes frequently for parents.

About the Writer

• • • • • •

KATHLEEN MOLONEY has written or cowritten books on many subjects, including baseball *(Baseball by the Rules)*, etiquette *(Esquire Etiquette)*, ventriloquism *(Ventriloquism for the Total Dummy)*, and health *(40 Plus for Women)*. She lives in New York City.

Series Introduction

● ● ● ● ● ●

What do children need to learn about themselves and the world around them if they are to realize their potential? What can parents do to facilitate their children's emotional, physical, and intellectual growth?

For more than a generation, Children's Television Workshop, creators of *Sesame Street*, has asked these questions and has conducted extensive research to uncover the answers. We have gathered together some of the best minds in child development, health, and communication. We have studied what experts around the world are doing to nurture this generation. And, most important, we have worked with children and parents to get direct feedback on what it means to be a productive and fulfilled family member in our rapidly changing world. We recognize that there are no simple solutions to the inherent complexities of child rearing and that in most situations, there are no single answers that apply to all families. Thus, we do not offer a "how-to" approach to being a parent. Rather, we present facts where information will help each of you make appropriate decisions, and we offer strategies for finding solutions to the varied concerns of individual families.

The development of the CTW Family Living Series is a natural outgrowth of our commitment to share what we have learned with parents and others who care for today's children. It is hoped that the information presented here will make the job of parenting a little easier—and more fun.

Contents

••••••

CONTENTS

CONTENTS

Preface

• • • • • •

These are trying times for parents who want to teach their children good eating habits. In nearly every family, there is at least one major *internal* obstacle. You may be a single parent with an outside job or career who comes racing home each day, tired and hungry, to prepare supper for children who themselves may be cranky and hungry (or not hungry because they stuffed themselves with junk food all afternoon). Or you may be part of a two-parent family in which both of you have outside jobs, perhaps complicated by frequent out-of-town trips, business dinners, and other off-hour obligations. Either way, you find yourself relying more and more on take-out foods and factory-prepared meals that may not be nutritionally ideal. On many nights, you may abandon any thoughts of in-house meal preparation and simply take the whole family out for a fast-food or restaurant supper.

In still other families—probably a majority these days—the family meal has fallen on hard times, enjoyed perhaps once a week on Sunday afternoon. Between professional and social obligations of the parents and lessons and sports activities pursued by the children, there is hardly a night when the whole family is home at the same time to sit down to a meal together.

Then there are the myriad *external* obstacles. They start with the plethora of television commercials for cereals and snacks that are nutritionally wanting. Of course, the Madison Avenue techniques that sell them convince your children that life is not worth living unless they start the day with a heavily fortified cereal that may be 50 percent sugar. But there is no one to fortify *you* against the screaming supermarket scene when you try to deny your children these "nutritious" wonders.

Even before your children can give voice to advertising influences, you may have to relinquish their care and feeding to babysitters, housekeepers, or day-care operators, whose primary goals may be to please the child, not the parents, and to save money. Sugary drinks are far less costly than pure fruit juices. And three-packages-for-a-dollar cookies go a lot further than fresh fruit. It's certainly easier (and often cheaper) to toss a hot dog in a pan or prepare packaged noodles and cheese (loaded with salt, fat, and additives) than to make a wholesome main-dish soup or spaghetti with nutritious sauce from scratch.

Once your children go off to school, nutrition can fall even further by the wayside. Despite much sound and fury, school lunches in most areas are a nutritional disgrace. Most schools provide foods that are least expensive (including free government-surplus commodities like fat- and salt-laden cheese) and that result in the least waste. In other words, they give kids what kids will eat—mainly foods that mimic those sold in fast-food establishments. And for the concerned parent who sends a child to school with a brown-bag lunch, there is the behind-the-scenes trading to contend with: The apple you so conscientiously provided may be exchanged for a brownie or a bag of chips, or the turkey sandwich traded for bologna.

The older children get, the less control you have over their meals and snacks and the worse their nutritional habits are likely to become. What is a parent to do?

You can start by reading this book. It is a highly informative yet simple guide to fostering nutritious eating habits from the day your baby is born until your child is through high school and presumably old enough to assume responsibility for the nutritional quality of his or her meals. The book is filled with practical advice, such as how to cope with picky eaters, how to feed children who have allergies or illnesses, how to recognize eating disorders, what to do about adverse reactions to food, when to seek nutrition counseling, and how to prepare family meals when you're hardly ever home. Of course, the book also provides the basics of good nutrition for children of varying ages and circumstances (you will discover, for example, just how little food a small child actually requires to be well nourished) and offers tips on such common parental concerns as how to get children to try new foods and what to do about relatives and caretakers who ply children with nutritionally undesirable foods and snacks.

You may be wondering, "How important is all this anyway?" The answer is, "It's very important." Although children are very resilient and seem to be able to bounce back readily from most noxious influences, studies strongly suggest that their eating habits can affect their ability to concentrate and learn, their energy level and self-control, their resistance to ordinary illnesses, and their athletic ability, as well as their overall stamina and growth. For example, children who try to get through the morning without breakfast tend to have trouble concentrating and learning and are more disruptive in the classroom during the hour or so before lunch.

Furthermore, as medical researchers delve into the antecedents of the nation's leading killer diseases, they are finding more and more that what and how we eat in childhood sets the stage for good health or bad in our adult years.

After all, parental responsibility goes beyond the teen years. If you love your children and are concerned about their welfare, you should care about how healthy and happy they will be when they reach your present age. As research evidence accumulates, it is becoming apparent that the nutritional stage for heart disease, high blood pressure, obesity, and certain cancers is set in childhood. We would all be better off if we grew up consuming foods that were relatively low in fat, salt, and sugar and rich in dietary fiber. And we would have a far easier time at weight control as adults if we didn't leave adolescence with an overaccumulation of permanent fat cells that are constantly asking us to fill them up.

Even for those diet-related conditions that may not be rooted in youth, the eating habits established early in life are the ones people tend to pursue into adulthood. It is far easier to start out eating properly than to have to try to make a switch as an adult. If, for example, your children start out eating treats that are low in sugar, they are less likely to crave overly sweetened, commercially prepared "goodies." I knew I had won that battle when, after years of providing my sons with minimally sweetened home-made muffins and cookies they rejected a piece of rich chocolate cake with the comment, "Yuck, Mommy, this is too sweet." And by never having soft drinks in the house, I managed to get my sons to the age of ten before either could finish an entire can of cola. Even as teenagers out with their friends, they more often choose milk, juice, or water to drink than a sugary soft drink.

One of the best ways to get kids to eat properly is to do so yourself. Children learn by example. If they see that their parents never leave the house without breakfast, they will be less inclined to do so themselves. If they see their parents eating fruit rather than cookies or cake for dessert and snacks, they will be more likely to choose fruit themselves. Of course, it helps a great deal if the house is well stocked with nutritionally desirable foods and devoid of empty-calorie items, except, perhaps, on special occasions. A hungry child will eat what's there. If there's a bowl of fruit on the table and no cookies in the jar, the fruit is what will get eaten.

Do you wonder how you can possibly fit good nutrition into your already overscheduled life? You do it just the way you accomplish anything else you consider important—by making it a priority, by making a commitment to it. Always keep in mind that the way you fuel your body and your children's bodies largely determines how well their bodies will run, both now and in the future. I don't pretend that it is easy these days to make good nutrition a way of life, but I do know that it's important, important enough for you to sacrifice something else to make it happen. That is a challenge all of us parents face these days, but I am certain it is a challenge worth meeting. Now, let the *Parents' Guide to Feeding Your Kids Right* help you do it.

JANE BRODY

A Few Words About Pronouns

• • • • • •

The child fell off *his* bike.'' Or how about ''The child fell off *her* bike''? Then again we could say, ''The child fell off *his or her* bike.'' How to deal with pronouns?

If you are a regular reader of *Sesame Street Magazine Parents' Guide,* you know that our policy is to alternate the use of gender-related pronouns. In one paragraph we say *his;* in the following one we use *her.* In a book, that specific policy is not quite as practical—there are just too many paragraphs—but it works in a general way by alternating chapters and special sections.

PART I

......

Food and the Body

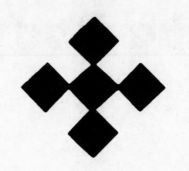

Introduction to Part I

• • • • • •

Keeping fit has become a national obsession. At least we *think* about good health quite a bit. *Doing* something about our health and the health of our children is harder because there's a lot to know before we can begin to change our habits. Some of us go to extremes in our diets, needlessly depriving ourselves of the simple pleasures of eating because we're convinced that certain foods are just plain bad. Or we stick to a very limited diet, convinced that certain foods hold the key to good health and long life. As with most things, the truth lies somewhere in between.

Eating healthfully is easier today than it's ever been. Foods from all food groups are available year-round; many foods are vitamin-enriched and -fortified to boost their value; and the latest research confirms that no single food and no one category of food is inherently good or bad. We've also learned that childhood eating habits can lay the groundwork for adult health—and that the way children learn to think about food can be as important to their well-being as the foods they eat.

In this section, we'll begin by looking at how we feel about food, and we'll discuss the wonderful variety of foods that constitute a healthful diet.

CHAPTER ONE

· · · · · ·

How Do We Feel About Food?

Everyone approaches food and eating differently, and most of our ideas are formed by the eating experiences we had when we were growing up. For some people, food is equated with warm and comfortable feelings; like a parent's love, a good meal can make all things right again. For others, food is a reason for family and friends to gather; the food is important but not as important as the socializing. Still others were taught that food is a reward for accomplishments or a balm for disappointments: getting a good report card, sitting still through a haircut, or losing the big game. And then there are those for whom the memories of mealtime stresses during childhood have made food the object of virtual dread; it's hard to look forward to mealtime when you're sure that someone is going to start an argument as soon as the soup is served.

Such memories and feelings dictate many of our feelings about food and eating. Perhaps by questioning our own approaches to food we can better consider specific messages we are sending our children:

- **Is the table a pleasant place to be or is it the stage for family squabbles?** Obviously, the more pleasant the atmosphere, the more likely it is that your family will enjoy mealtime.

- **Who does the talking at the table? Do you find yourself directing what and how food should be eaten more than discussing the day's events or other nonfood topics?** Remember, the dinner table is a great place to get to know your kids—and for them to get to know you, too.

- **Do you encourage your child to try new foods—even ones you think he may not like?** The key word here is *encourage*. If kids aren't forced to eat something new, they'll be more willing to try later.

- **Do you insist that your child finish everything on his plate before leaving the table?** It helps to remember that eating should be a way to satisfy hunger, not a chore or a challenge.

- **Do you withhold dessert if your child has not finished his main course?** Try allowing smaller main-course portions, followed by smaller dessert portions. Variety is important in the enjoyment of a meal.

- **Do you allow before-meal or after-meal snacking?** Too much snacking will interfere with mealtime appetites. You may want to consider rescheduling meals to coincide better with hunger pangs.

- **Do you encourage your child's active participation in meal planning and preparation?** Children who are involved in planning are much more likely to enjoy the end product.

- **Do you enjoy mealtime?** Share the good feeling with your kids!

Think about the messages you send through your own behavior and decide if these are the behaviors you want your child to imitate. As you and your children gather around your table, it is important to remember that you can do more than serve healthful foods; you can instill healthy ideas about food and mealtime.

What Constitutes a Healthy Notion of Food?

Children who grow up with healthy attitudes toward food have certain childhood eating experiences in common:

- They learned that the dinner table was a pleasant place to be, not a battleground where they and their parents tested one another's wills.

- They learned that food was an antidote to physical hunger, not an emotional reward or a source of punishment.

- They learned that it was okay to leave food on their plates rather than to force down unwanted foods. (So that food won't be wasted, they were encouraged to take small portions and to come back for more if they wanted to.)

- They were encouraged to try new foods but were not forced to eat regular-size portions of new or disliked foods.

- Their parents understood that food quirks (such as refusing to eat a food that had touched another food) and food jags (refusing anything but tuna fish for weeks on end, for example) were normal stages of development for many children. Thus, their parents did not attempt to force a change in these temporary behaviors.

- They learned to enjoy a variety of foods, never learning that some foods were inherently good while others were

7

inherently bad. Since no foods, such as sweets, were "off limits," they didn't learn to place too high a value on these foods. Likewise, since no foods, such as spinach, were used as bargaining chips to earn dessert, they didn't learn to devalue any food or food group as "what you have to eat in order to get the good stuff."

- They knew they were loved for more than their ability to please their parents. Thus, "eating right" (or getting the best grades or being the most popular) was not a central focus of their lives.

- They had parents who set good examples by eating healthfully themselves, not by lecturing on the need for good nutrition.

The Family Meal in an Eat-and-Run Era

For many families today, the ritual of gathering around the dinner table for a home-cooked meal is a wished-for but not-always-possible occurrence. What can busy parents do to instill good nutritional values, a positive attitude toward eating, and even some table manners in their children when everyone is on the run? Some suggestions:

- At least twice a week, meet for regular at-home meals. Concentrate on catch-up conversation. The food doesn't have to be fancy, but the atmosphere should be as pleasant as possible.

- Enlist the kids' help in grocery shopping and meal preparation. These occasions allow you to discuss why you choose the foods you do.

- Once in a while, meet your child for lunch. Kids love having a parent's complete attention, which isn't always possible with the daily distractions at home.

- Include an "I-love-you" note in your child's lunchbox or in the refrigerator on top of his afternoon snack if you aren't home yourself to give an after-school hug. (Include such notes on the hall mirror or child's pillow, too. After all, feeding them isn't the only way to show love—and eating isn't the only way for children to feel loved!)

- Limit snacking during TV time—and turn off the TV during dinner time.

- Be polite to your children, not just at the dinner table, but in general. Let them know you expect the same courtesy from them.

● ●

Advice from Parents

Readers of *Sesame Street Magazine Parents' Guide* were asked:

Do you think it's important for the whole family to eat meals together, or do you prefer to feed your children separately?

Their responses:

"I do not agree with feeding children separately. This does not allow for a family to experience conversation with all its members and usually means more work for the parent to fix a separate meal."

—Mary E. Kolb
East Greenbush, NY

"I feel very strongly about eating together as a family. We enjoy each other's company at the table. We have a special meal night once every two weeks where my three- and four-year-olds pick out their favorite meal and put it on the menu. They really enjoy it—especially when my four-year-old slipped ice cream on the menu. We all laughed at first. Then we decided to take her advice. We went to our favorite ice cream parlor and loaded the ice cream down with as much nutrition as possible: nuts, bananas, strawberries, and cherries. Then we relaxed and enjoyed one of our best meals ever!"

—Sandy Butze
Riverside, CA

"Mealtime is a great time to let the children do most of the talking and the parents listen!"

—Jeannie Pagnotta
Newcastle, OK

"I believe it's very important for families to eat together. When our oldest child was one, we started a tradition of 'Friday Night Picnic.' We usually have pizza or some other special dinner. We all look forward to our picnics, which usually take place on the living-room floor.

The only time the children are fed separately is when we're having a party and want to share time with our friends."

—Sally Hartley
Salix, LA

"It is important for the whole family to eat meals together. My three-year-old daughter is learning correct table manners and how to talk socially. She learns about her father's and my day, and we, in turn, learn about hers."

—Laura Skaggs
Louisville, KY

"I feel it is important for parents to spend precious time together alone, but mealtime is for talking and laughing with *all* family members. Of course, some functions do call for the children to eat separately, and I feel it will not affect them."

—Kathleen L. Tansy
West Chester, PA

"We feel it is important for children to observe the proper way to eat and to try to have at least one meal [a day] with the whole family together. We have discussions on the day's events and try to compliment the children and each other when we use proper manners. There are times, however, when Mom and Dad need time alone, and then the dining room becomes 'McConnell's Restaurant' for the children. I take orders for food and drinks and they enjoy being 'grown up.' Later, my husband and I have our dinner together, enjoying each other's company and a meal, such as fish or something gourmet, which the children might complain about eating."

—Tom and Laura McConnell
Jewett, OH

"Just as nutritionists suggest offering your child a variety of foods, I think the same goes for offering a variety of changes in the dinner atmosphere. Most nights, having dinner together as a family is very rewarding for all of those concerned. But letting your children eat without you on occasion

teaches them to have some responsibility and that you trust them to handle the situation by themselves."
—Gaye L. Sanders
Hastings, MI

"Mealtime is very important for our family to spend together. We have also found that if the kids help in preparing the meal, they feel more involved and they eat better. Our three-year-old is one mean salad maker, and our two-year-old can set a beautiful table."
—Donnita Nesbit Fisher
Dallas, TX

"We think it's quite important for children to be at the table with adults, but after a long day's work my husband and I have a need to be alone together for a little while, too. At our house, we've arranged it this way: About twice a week the children are fed before us. My husband relaxes by himself with the day's mail or TV news while I sit with Jennifer and David. Later on, when the kids are in bed, we have a meal by ourselves. One night a week, I work late and my husband feeds the kids entirely on his own—another ritual they enjoy. The other nights, we eat together. Whatever the routine, we try to insist on *sitting down,* not grazing."
—Anna Hart
Alexandria, VA

"Dinnertime is the one time we all touch base, catch up, share jokes and stories, and yes, we even argue. Our dinners last at least forty-five minutes to an hour, and we have a good time together. Everyone except the baby is responsible for either preparing the meal or cleaning up afterwards."
—Jeanine Chatt
Lockport, NY

CHAPTER TWO

······

What Do the Words Mean? A Dictionary of Nutrition-Related Terms

We all know about the need for good nutrition. It's just a matter of eating all the right proteins, carbohydrates, vitamins, and minerals every day, right? That's true, of course. But just what are proteins? How are vitamins different from one another—and where do we get them?

The primary needs of the body are met by eating a combination of foods containing the basic nutrients: proteins, carbohydrates, and fats; vitamins and minerals; and water and fiber. Proteins, carbohydrates, and fats provide the body with energy, while vitamins and minerals help maintain chemical balances. Fiber is important for digestion, and water is vital for all the body's functions. Most foods contain a combination of nutrients, and there is no single food that must be consumed and no single food that must be avoided. A good diet for both adults and children is one that includes foods containing proper proportions of all the nutrients we need, and the best way to achieve this is to eat a variety of foods.

The mix of needed nutrients doesn't remain exactly the same throughout our lives, either. At different stages of our lives, our bodies' needs are different, and it's important not to confuse the needs of adults' bodies with the needs of growing children's bodies. (The particular needs of children at various stages are discussed in chapters 5 through 10.) But, no matter what our age, each of us needs a diet that balances the consumption of proteins, carbohydrates, and fats. Such a diet will, quite naturally, fulfill our need for vitamins and minerals and will contain the right proportions of fiber and water. Now let's look at those fundamental food components.

Proteins

Protein is found in every cell of the body and is involved in thousands of the body's activities, including digestion and metabolism. The body uses protein to form and maintain tissues and cells, to regulate the balance of water, acids, and bases in the system, and to carry nutrients in and out of the cells.

Protein-rich foods include red meats, poultry, fish, eggs, milk-based products, legumes, and nuts.

The body also uses protein to make antibodies, which play a major role in combating invading substances, particularly the bacteria that cause disease. Proteins transport oxygen and nutrients in the blood and are important in the formation of scar tissue and in blood clotting. They also have a prominent place in the composition of enzymes, substances that help control the chemical processes of the body. In short, proteins are indispensable to the functioning of the body.

Proteins are composed of chains of amino acids (called "the building blocks of protein") which contain nitrogen.

The quality of protein in a given food is determined by the amount and kinds of the amino acids it contains. Animal proteins, such as meat, eggs, fish, and milk, contain *all* of the essential amino acids in the ideal proportions. These proteins are capable of maintaining body cells and promoting growth, and for this reason they are considered high-quality proteins. (Being animal in nature, they are also closer in composition to the human body than vegetable proteins.) Vegetable or plant proteins contain all the amino acids, but not in the ideal proportions, and, as a result, they are less complete. These less-complete proteins must be eaten in combination with other foods (combining rice with beans, for example), to create the right balance to fulfill the body's many needs. Thus, a vegetarian can indeed consume all the needed proteins—provided that she eats vegetable proteins in the right combinations.

While animal protein is important, the theory that more is better doesn't really hold. If it did, most Americans would be perfect specimens. The truth is, contrary to decades of cultural training that have instilled in us the notion that animal protein ranks above all other nutrients, the body actually needs only a limited amount of animal protein, provided that the diet contains enough calories for growth and maintenance from other food sources. For both children and adults, the amount of protein in the diet should translate into approximately 15 percent of the day's caloric intake.

Carbohydrates

Carbohydrates provide the primary source of energy for the body. Foods high in carbohydrate content include fruits, vegetables, grains, and grain products such as bread, pasta, and cereals. Cookies, cakes, and pies, too, are high-carbohydrate foods.

There are two basic types of carbohydrates: complex carbohydrates, also known as *starches,* and simple carbohydrates, commonly called *sugars.* To confuse matters even more, both kinds of carbohydrates break down into forms of sugar in the body.

The complex carbohydrates—such as those found in vegetables, fruits, and grains, which come in "nature's packages"—are considerably more nutritious than simple carbohydrates such as the table sugar found in sweetened desserts. Fruits, grains, and vegetables contain protein, vitamins, and minerals in addition to sugars and starches, but candy and other sweets do not; that's why the nutrition they provide, which comes mostly from sugar, is occasionally referred to as "empty calories." Fruits, vegetables, and grains also contain an important non-nutrient: fiber. Fiber doesn't provide energy (it has no calories), but it is nevertheless important to the overall diet and the functioning of the body, especially to the digestive system.

....

CONSUMER TIP: We often choose "wheat" bread over "white" bread, assuming that the darker loaf is the healthier one. This is true only when the wheat is *whole* wheat. White bread, too, is made from wheat, and loaves that are marked *wheat* but not *whole wheat* are darker simply because caramel coloring has been added in the processing.
....

16

The calories in all fruits, vegetables, and grains are derived principally from carbohydrates, although these foods may also contain protein, and even fat.

For years, starches such as potatoes, rice, and breads have been looked upon as fattening, definitely to be avoided if you're concerned about your weight. Ounce for ounce, however, these complex carbohydrates are an excellent source of low-fat, high-fiber energy and other nutrients. What's more, they are filling, and they come in all shapes and sizes. Perhaps best of all, kids love them.

A healthful diet for both adults and children derives about 55 percent of its calories from carbohydrates, primarily complex carbohydrates.

Fats

All fats are a combination of saturated and unsaturated fatty acids, but in certain foods there is a preponderance of one type of fatty acid over another, which is why we call a fat *saturated* or *unsaturated*.

Fats are our most concentrated dietary source of energy, which is another way of saying "highest in calories." Fat supplies about 9 calories of energy per gram (compared with 4 calories per gram for carbohydrates and protein), but it does a lot more for the body besides fuel it. It provides essential fatty acids that the body cannot make, carries fat-soluble vitamins, forms a part of cell membranes, and makes it possible for the body to get energy from carbohydrates and proteins. Fat deposits in the body insulate it and protect vital organs. And most important to our taste buds, fats improve the flavor and texture of many foods.

Foods that are rich in fat include meat, cheese, butter, and vegetable oils.

....

CONSUMER TIP: The word *light* (or *lite*) on a processed food does not necessarily mean *dietetic*. The word simply means that there is less fat (and fewer calories) in these versions of the product than in other versions of the same product. The item may still be a high-fat food.

....

Many of the fats found in foods and in the body are known as *triglycerides*. There are many different forms of triglycerides, but they are all made up of glycerol and free fatty acids. Fatty acids are chains of carbon atoms, two to more than twenty atoms long. Their length and saturation help determine the characteristics of the fat. Saturation refers to the ratio of carbon atoms to hydrogen atoms.

When a fatty acid holds all the hydrogen atoms it can handle, it is termed *saturated*. These saturated fatty acids are found primarily in animal products—red meat, eggs, butter, and other whole-milk dairy products—but there are a few vegetable oils that are heavily saturated, too: coconut oil, palm oil, and palm kernel oil. Some fat you can see (just take a look at the edge of a steak or a pat of butter), but some is invisible.

Much of the concern about the cause-and-effect relationship between heart disease and dietary fat focuses on saturated fatty acids, the ''bad fats,'' which can deposit substances that clog arteries and obstruct blood flow to the heart, which can result in a heart attack or angina.

Unsaturated fats—the ''good fats''—contain fatty acids to which more hydrogen atoms can be attached. Unsaturated fatty acids are divided into two types: monounsaturated and polyunsaturated.

Monounsaturated fatty acids are found in some animal fats

and a number of vegetable fats. Olive oil, peanut oil, and avocados are especially good sources of monounsaturated fatty acids.

Polyunsaturated fatty acids are found primarily in vegetable fats; oils made from corn, cottonseeds, safflowers, sunflowers, and soybeans are the most common sources of polyunsaturated fatty acids.

....

CONSUMER TIP: Knowing that Americans are anxious about the level of cholesterol in their foods, some manufacturers advertise *cholesterol-free* breads, cereals, and other grain products. While this is not false advertising, it is somewhat misleading, since grains are naturally cholesterol-free.
....

Cholesterol is found *only* in animal tissue and is essential for the development of the nervous system. It is also thought to be a leading culprit in the development of arterial heart disease. (In some people, cholesterol forms deposits along artery walls, constricting blood flow.) Both monounsaturated and polyunsaturated fatty acids in the diet in moderate amounts seem to lower blood-cholesterol levels, while saturated fatty acids tend to raise blood-cholesterol levels. While limiting the intake of saturated fats in an adult's diet is a good thing to do, reducing a young child's fat intake too much can be hazardous. Children *need* some fat in their diets to give them the energy they need to play and the calories they need to promote growth. Thus, serving low-fat dairy products to young children should not be done.

Still, the issue of kids and cholesterol should not be ignored. Recent studies show that one out of every four American children between the ages of five and eighteen has a higher-than-ideal level of blood cholesterol, and one out of twenty has what's considered a very high level. Some studies show that a child with high levels of cholesterol may take the problem into adulthood. The American Heart Association urges that adults and older children (grade-school age and teens) limit the fat intake in their diets to 30 percent of the calories consumed daily, with 10 percent each from saturated, monounsaturated, and polyunsaturated fats. The American Academy of Pediatrics recommends that the daily diet of children under five should be 35 percent fat, reflecting the greater energy needs of young children. If, however, there is a history of high cholesterol and heart disease in your family, the Academy recommends that you have your child's cholesterol level tested regularly from the age of two. You should also be particularly watchful of the fat content of your child's diet and should encourage your child to restrict her fat intake as she gets older. There is another benefit in lowering fat intake in older children: It will help them establish eating habits now that will serve them well when they get older and the need for eating a low-fat diet becomes more important.

Vitamins

Vitamins help the body process proteins, carbohydrates, and fats. Certain vitamins also play a role in the formation of blood cells, hormones, genetic material, and chemicals of the nervous system, and as an aid to enzymes. Vitamins also help chemical reactions in the body to occur. Vitamins can be divided roughly into two categories: those that are soluble in *water* and those that are soluble in *fat*. The water-soluble vitamins—vitamin C and the eight B vitamins—must be consumed daily, since the body only has moderate means of storing most of them.

The fat-soluble vitamins—A, D, E, and K—are absorbed with the fats in the diet and can be stored for days, weeks, or even months by the body. Despite their long "shelf life," it's important to eat foods that contain fat-soluble vitamins regularly (a few times a week), to ensure that no vitamin depletion takes place. Besides, foods rich in these vitamins are good sources of other nutrients.

....

CONSUMER TIP: Some processed foods are labeled *enriched*. Others are labeled *fortified*. What's the difference? Enriched foods contain vitamins in quantities above what is natural for that product. Fortified foods contain vitamins that do not naturally appear in that product.
....

The two vitamins we now hear most about are A and C. Vitamin A, found in fish oil, liver, leafy dark green and orange vegetables, and egg yolks, is responsible for maintaining healthy skin and mucous membranes and for forming bones and tooth enamel. Studies are being done to find out if vitamin A might also be useful in preventing cancers of the epithelial tissues, such as the lung and the bladder. For all of vitamin A's known and potentially desirable properties, however, vitamin-pill megadoses of this vitamin can be toxic. How much vitamin A do we need and where can we get it?

Recommended Dietary Allowance
for Vitamin A

	Age	International Units (IUs)
Children	6 mo.–3	1,600
	4–6	2,000
	7–10	2,800
Women	11+	4,000
Men	11+	5,000
Pregnant women	—	5,000
Lactating women	—	6,000

Some Sources of Vitamin A

Food	Serving Size	IUs/Serving
Liver, beef	3 oz, fried	45,400
Carrots	½ cup, diced, boiled	7,900
Apricots, dried	1 medium raw	7,600
Leafy green vegetables	½ cup	3,300+
Winter squash	½ cup, cooked	4,300
Sweet potatoes	1 medium, baked	9,200
Cantaloupe	½ melon or 1 cup, cubed	5,400
Broccoli	½ cup, cooked	1,900
Lettuce, green leaves	1 cup, chopped	1,000
Tomatoes	1 medium, raw	1,000
Milk	1 cup	275
Eggs	1 yolk	300
Butter/Margarine	1 tsp	150
Cream	Light, 4 tbsp	450

Source: Adapted from *Nutrition and Health,* by Kathleen Oliver Carpenter and Doris Howes Calloway, copyright © 1981 by Saunders College Publishing, reproduced by permission of the publisher.

Vitamin C, also known as *ascorbic acid*, is found in abundance in citrus fruits and leafy green vegetables. This vitamin has been said to be capable of warding off colds, flu, and even cancer. Controlled studies have not yet borne this theory out, however, although cold symptoms are thought to be reduced somewhat in those ingesting large quantities of the vitamin. Two of vitamin C's normal functions in the body are to promote collagen formation (collagen is the "cementing" agent that holds the cells together) and to enhance the absorption of the minerals iron and calcium. It has also been shown to block the formation of nitrosamines, the cancer-causing substances that are found naturally in the body and that accumulate as a result of eating nitrate- and nitrite-treated foods (primarily processed and cured meats). How much vitamin C do we need and where can we get it?

Recommended Dietary Allowance for Vitamin C

	(Mg)
Infants 0–1 year	35
Children 1–10 years	45
11–14 years	50
Persons 15 years old and older	60
Pregnant women	80
Lactating women	100

Sources of Vitamin C

Food	Serving Size	*Mg/Serving
Fruits		
Apples, pears, peaches	1 cup	7
Blueberries	1 cup	20
Cantaloupe	½ of 5-inch melon	90
Sweet cherries		7
Grapefruit	½ medium	44
Juice		93
Grapes	10	2
Oranges	1	66
Juice	1 cup	110
Papaya	1 cup ½-inch cubes	78
Strawberries	1 cup, raw	88
Watermelon	1 4×8-inch wedge	50
Vegetables		
Bean sprouts (mung)	1 cup, raw	20
Broccoli, chopped	1 cup, cooked	105
Brussels sprouts	1 cup, cooked	130
Cabbage, green or red	1 cup, cooked	48
Cauliflower	1 cup, cooked	72
Cucumber slices	9 small pieces	3
Greens		
Kale (no stems or midribs)	1 cup cooked (from raw)	102
Turnip (no stems or midribs)	1 cup cooked (from raw)	67

Food	Serving Size	*Mg/Serving
Lettuce	1 cup, shredded	6
Peppers, sweet	1 whole, raw	94
Potatoes	1 large, baked	31
Spinach	1 cup raw	28
	1 cup cooked	45
Squash, all kinds	1 cup, cooked	24
Tomatoes	1 medium raw	28
Juice	1 cup	39

*Greens prepared from the frozen product have approximately half the vitamin C of those separated from stems and cooked from the raw state.

Source: From *Nutrition and Health,* by Kathleen Oliver Carpenter and Doris Howes Calloway, copyright © 1981 by Saunders College Publishing, reproduced by permission of the publisher.

Where to Find Other Vitamins in Food

Vitamin	Where to Find It	Why We Need It
Vitamin D	fortified milk, egg yolk, tuna, salmon, margarine (vitamin D is also found in sunlight.)	• helps body build and maintain teeth and bones • helps body absorb calcium and phosphorus
Vitamin E	vegetable oils and margarine, leafy green vegetables	• helps body create and maintain red blood cells
Vitamin K	The bacteria in the intestinal tract provide all the vitamin K we need.	• aids in blood clotting • maintains bones
Vitamin B_1 (thiamine)	whole-grain and enriched breads and cereals, pork, poultry, organ meats, peas, lima beans, dried beans, brewer's yeast	• helps body use carbohydrates • aids muscle coordination • maintains nervous system and heart
Vitamin B_2 (riboflavin)	leafy green vegetables, liver, meat, enriched breads and cereals, milk, eggs, yeast, seeds, and nuts	• develops and maintains healthy body tissue and skin

Vitamin	Where to Find It	Why We Need It
Niacin	liver, poultry, meat, fish, eggs, whole-grain and enriched cereals, bread, and pasta, nuts, dried legumes	• works with other B vitamins to use energy in cells
Vitamin B_6	whole-grain cereals, wheat germ, meat, liver, vegetables (especially potatoes), dried beans, bananas	• develops healthy teeth and gums and red blood cells • aids in the formation of some proteins • helps the body use fats • aids functioning of the nervous system
B_{12} (cobalamin)	liver, poultry, meat, eggs, milk	• aids functioning of the nervous system • helps body create and maintain red blood cells
Folacin	liver, kidneys, dark leafy green vegetables, wheat germ, dried legumes, yeast, orange juice, nuts	• works with vitamin B_{12} to form genetic material • helps to form hemoglobin in red blood cells

Vitamin	Where to Find It	Why We Need It
Pantothenic acid	liver, kidneys, whole-grain cereals and bread, nuts, eggs, dark green vegetables	• helps metabolize carbohydrates, proteins, and fats • aids in formation of hormones and nerve-regulating chemicals
Biotin	egg yolk, kidneys, yeast, liver	• aids in creation of fatty acids • releases energy from carbohydrates

Minerals

Like vitamins, minerals are necessary to keep the body functioning. Also like vitamins, they are found primarily in the foods we eat, and they perform a wide variety of functions. Eating a well-balanced diet will ensure that we get most of the minerals we need, but there are two minerals that we should be particularly conscientious about consuming in adequate amounts: calcium and iron.

Calcium

Calcium, which is present in bones, teeth, blood, and soft tissues, plays a role in controlling heartbeat, transmitting nerve messages, contracting muscles, clotting blood, and activating enzymes. The average person's body contains about 2 percent calcium; thus, if you weigh 150 pounds, 3 pounds of that is calcium. How much calcium do we need to consume every day and where can we get it?

Recommended Dietary Allowances of Calcium

	Age	(Mg)
Infants	0–6 months	360
	6 months–1 year	540
Children	1–10 years	800
	11–18 years	1,200
Most Adults		800
Pregnant and Nursing Women		1,200

Sources of Calcium

	Mg/Serving
Sesame seeds, whole, ¼ cup	348
Milk, 8-oz. glass	285
Salmon, red, canned with bones, ⅖ cup	259
Sardines, canned in oil, 2 fish drained	174
Cheese, cheddar, 1 oz	225
Leafy vegetables, avg. ½ cup, cooked	140
Ice cream, plain, avg. ¾ cup	123
Molasses, medium, 2 tbsp	116
Broccoli, ⅔ cup	88
Baked beans, ½ cup, canned with	
molasses	82
tomato sauce	70
Orange, 1 medium	62

	Mg/Serving
Cottage cheese, 2 round tbsp	52
String beans, ⅔ cup, cooked	50
Parsnips, ½ cup, cooked	44
Lima beans, ½ cup, cooked	38

Source: From *Nutrition and Health,* by Kathleen Oliver Carpenter and Doris Howes Callo-way, copyright © 1981 by Saunders College Publishing, reproduced by permission of the publisher.

The absorption of calcium into the system is dependent on a number of factors in addition to the amount eaten. Certain vitamins, such as C and D, play a role in calcium absorption, as does lactose, the sugar in milk. Your body is also capable of absorbing more calcium from calcium-rich foods when it needs extra amounts. For instance, growing children and pregnant women, who have a special need for calcium, absorb more of the available calcium from the foods they eat than others do.

Iron

In contrast to calcium, iron is found only in trace amounts in most foods. Iron is essential to the working of all cells, especially the muscle cells and the red blood cells, which carry oxygen. When the blood doesn't have enough iron, oxygen is not efficiently carried through the body, and we end up feeling tired and run down. The official term for this run-down feeling is *iron-deficiency anemia,* and it's the most common nutritional deficiency in the country today. The best way to prevent it is to eat foods that are rich in iron. Once again, eating foods rich in vitamin C along with iron-rich foods increases the body's ability to absorb iron. How much iron do we need and where can we get it?

Recommended Dietary Allowances for Iron

	Age	(Mg)
Infants	0–6 months	10
	6 months–1 year	15
Children	1–3 years	15
	4–10 years	10
	11–18 years	18
Men	19+ years	10
Women	19–50 years	18
	51+ years	10
	Pregnant	Iron supplements recommended
	Nursing	Iron supplements recommended for 2–3 months to replenish stores depleted by pregnancy

Source: From *Nutrition and Health,* by Kathleen Oliver Carpenter and Doris Howes Calloway, copyright © 1981 by Saunders College Publishing, reproduced by permission of the publisher.

Eating foods rich in iron is the first step in getting iron into the system. The second is to increase the amount that is absorbed by the body so that it can be used; the "bioavailability" of iron is as important as the amount consumed. This is where the importance of eating a balanced diet is seen most clearly. There are two kinds of iron: *heme* and *nonheme*. Heme iron is the kind most easily absorbed by the body. About 40 percent of the iron in animal meats is heme iron, and the rest is nonheme iron. All of the iron in vegetables and grains is nonheme iron. If you eat meat, fish, or poultry, along with a vitamin C-rich food such as a tomato or a potato or half a grapefruit at a meal, the amount of iron absorbed is greater.

Some Sources of Iron

	Serving Size	Mg/Serving
Liver, beef	3 oz, fried	7.5
Liver, calf	3 oz, fried	12.1
Liver, chicken	½ cup, chopped	6.0
Hamburger	4 oz, raw	2.6
Pork chop	1 medium	2.7
Beans, baked	½ cup, canned	2.5
Beans, lima	½ cup, cooked	2.2
Peas	½ cup, frozen or canned	1.5
Peanut butter	1 tbsp	0.6
Green (spinach, mustard greens, etc.)	½ cup, cooked	0.8–2.0
Molasses, medium	1 tbsp	1.2
Molasses, blackstrap	1 tbsp	3.2

Additional dietary sources of iron include iron-fortified cereal and bread; dried fruits; oysters, sardines, scallops, shrimp, and tuna; and poultry.

Source: From *Nutrition and Health,* by Kathleen Oliver Carpenter and Doris Howes Calloway, copyright © 1981 by Saunders College Publishing, reproduced by permission of the publisher.

Water

Water is not considered a "food group," but it *is* the most essential substance that we consume. The body cannot exist without water. (The body of an adult is composed of about two-thirds water; a newborn is 85 percent water.) Every cell of the body depends on water to function, since it is the water in the blood that transports nutrients and oxygen to the cells and carries away waste products.

Water is present in all the foods we eat and drink. Even so, the best source of this life-sustaining material is a plain glass of water. Most nutritionists recommend that adults drink at least six 8-ounce glasses a day. The recommendation for children is four 8-ounce glasses a day. Infants' water needs are generally met through breast milk and formula.

Fiber

Fiber, like water, is not a nutrient, but it *is* essential to the normal functioning of the body. Foods high in complex carbohydrates—fruits, vegetables, and grains—are the best sources of dietary fiber. High-fiber foods are also the best-known protection against certain digestive diseases, including cancer of the colon. A well-balanced diet, which consists of 55 percent carbohydrates (most of which should be complex carbohydrates, such as fruits, vegetables, and whole-grain products), will contain all the fiber you or your child needs. Too much fiber can interfere with the absorption of calories. (The only time you might want to supplement fiber consumption is when suffering from chronic constipation.)

• •
What's a Calorie?

When the food we eat is processed, or "metabolized," by the body, one result is energy, or heat. This heat is measured in a unit known as the *calorie,* technically defined as the amount of heat needed to raise the temperature of 1 gram of water 1 degree centigrade. In food terms, that means the amount of food needed to produce 1 kilocalorie of energy (the *kilo* part is dropped in most references). Different foods produce more or less heat per serving, and thus they are referred to as having different caloric values. Fats supply about 9 calories per gram of weight; carbohydrates and protein supply approximately 4 calories per gram; water and fiber are calorie-free.

Calories have assumed an exaggerated importance in our weight-conscious society. To know the caloric value of a food without knowing the fat, protein, carbohydrate, and fiber content of that food is not to know it very well. It's like judging a person by her height and weight—while ignoring her character. Instead, calories must be understood in the context of a food's nutritional value and an individual's need for fuel. In other words, 1,000 calories of cake is not the nutritional equivalent of 1,000 calories of pasta. Thus, any family member looking to lose or gain weight by decreasing or increasing her caloric intake should concentrate on the quality, not the quantity, of foods' caloric value.

CHAPTER THREE

······

Meeting Your Family's Nutritional Needs

"One serving of protein?" Dad asked Mom, reading from the checklist.

"Check," she replied.

"Two servings of carbohydrates—the complex kind?"

"Check."

"Fats?"

"Check."

"Vitamins and minerals?"

"Check."

"Something high in fiber? And something to drink?"

"Check. Check."

"Okay, call the kids in. Dinner is served."

It's hard to imagine just what this family's meal looks like—and it can be equally difficult to figure out just what foods your family needs if they are to have a healthful diet. Since it's unlikely that your supermarket boasts a high-protein aisle or a complex-carbohydrate section, it might be helpful to translate the list of needed nutrients into a typical shopping expedition, answering the questions you might have along the way.

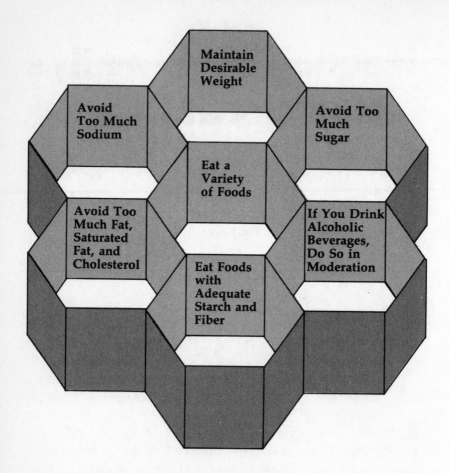

Maintain Desirable Weight

Avoid Too Much Sodium

Avoid Too Much Sugar

Eat a Variety of Foods

Avoid Too Much Fat, Saturated Fat, and Cholesterol

If You Drink Alcoholic Beverages, Do So in Moderation

Eat Foods with Adequate Starch and Fiber

GETTING THE RIGHT BALANCE

Good nutrition is a balancing act: Choosing foods with enough protein, vitamins, minerals, and fiber; but not too much fat, sodium, sugar, and alcohol. Also, energy (calorie) intake must be balanced with energy expended. The seven Dietary Guidelines, used together, can help you select a healthful diet.

Source: U.S. Department of Agriculture and U.S. Department of Health and Human Services, *Nutrition and Your Health: Dietary Guidelines for Americans,* August 1985.

High-Protein Foods

When shopping for foods high in protein, start in the meat and fish section of your supermarket. Then move on to the dairy section for more high-protein choices. You don't need to buy a lot—each adult in your family needs only 4 ounces per day. Kids need less—2 or 3 ounces per day, depending on their ages.

What kinds of meat are best?

Lean meats are far preferable to fatty meats. Choose cuts that can be baked, broiled, or steamed, rather than fried. To cut down on fat and cholesterol, without cutting down on meat, choose lean red meats, remove skin from poultry, and avoid prepackaged dinner meats and high-fat, processed luncheon meats. In an effort to cut down on fat, some people totally eliminate red meat in favor of poultry and fish. If you choose to do this, keep in mind that red meat provides more iron and zinc than either fish or poultry, so be sure to include other sources of these minerals, such as leafy green vegetables, beans, nuts, and seeds, in your shopping list.

My kids love hot dogs and bologna. Should I stop buying them?

Not necessarily. Look for luncheon meats that are made from low-fat turkey and that do not contain the additives nitrate or nitrite. Be careful, however, when serving hot dogs to young children because hot dogs are among the major causes of choking.

My children won't eat meat at all. What other high-protein foods can I serve them?

Try eggs, cottage cheese, or nonmeat protein sources in combination, such as macaroni and cheese, peanut butter on whole-grain bread, or beans and rice. With these combinations, you can be assured that your child (or any other vegetarian) will get his needed protein. Since iron from nonmeat sources is less well absorbed than the iron in meat, add a serving of a vitamin-C–rich food to meals that feature meat substitutes; this will increase the absorption of iron. If it's the texture rather than the meat itself that they don't like, try pureeing it or mixing it in with foods they do like.

Since eggs are high in cholesterol, shouldn't they be avoided?

Most adults and teens should limit their egg intake to one or two eggs per week. Children under the age of five, however, can eat an egg every day. It's one of the easiest ways to ensure that they're getting enough protein. And while most kids find eggs appealing, those who don't can eat egg-rich custard or other egg-laden foods.

● ●

Typical 1-Ounce Servings of High-Protein Foods

- A meatball 1 inch in diameter

- A hamburger 2 inches in diameter and ½-inch thick

- A 1-inch cube of stew meat

- A medium-size egg

- A slice of luncheon meat

- A 1-inch cube of cheese

- A slice of processed cheese

- ¼ cup of cottage cheese

- 2 tablespoons of peanut butter

- ½ cup dried peas or beans, cooked

Source: No-Nonsense Nutrition for Kids, by Jo-Ann Heslin and Annette B. Natow, published by McGraw-Hill, 1985/Pocket Books, 1986. Reprinted by permission.

High-Carbohydrate Foods

To shop for good sources of complex carbohydrates, begin in the produce aisle and then move on to the bakery section. You'll also find good sources of high-carbohydrate food in the packaged-goods and canned-goods sections.

Fruits and Vegetables

Choose a dark green, orange, or yellow fruit or vegetable three to five times a week for its vitamin-A value. Examples include spinach, broccoli, sweet potatoes, carrots, cantaloupe, mangoes, papayas, peaches, apricots, and watermelon. Spinach and carrots can easily be tucked into stews, spaghetti sauces, and casseroles. Fresh fruits and vegetables are usually the highest in nutritional value, but don't overlook frozen and canned varieties: They are economical, keep well, and provide good nutritional value. Canned fruits served with two tablespoons of syrup are a more than

acceptable alternative to pies, cakes, cookies, and candy—
and most kids like them.

One portion per day for both kids and adults should include a fruit rich in vitamin C, such as citrus fruits (and
juices), tomatoes, melons, and strawberries; or apple,
grape, and pineapple juices that are fortified with vitamin C.

Allow four ¼- to ⅓-cup portions per day for each preschool child and four ½-cup portions for everyone else.

**My kids won't touch green vegetables. Can they still eat
a well-balanced diet?**

Many young children don't like the bitter taste of green
vegetables, and it will do them no harm to skip them
until their palates are ready. Orange and yellow vegetables, particularly when served raw, are good substitute
sources of vitamin A and fiber. Fruits can take the place
of greens, too. Mangoes, for example, contain the same
amount of fiber and vitamin A per serving as spinach.
While not all foods will provide exact nutritional equiva-
lents, if kids eat a wide enough variety of foods, they'll
be fine. It's important to remember that greens are also
an important source of iron. If family members are not
eating enough iron-rich foods, they can get their needed
iron from canned fish or from iron-fortified cereals.

**My children won't eat whole fruits, but they love fruit
juices. Are fruit juices a good source of carbohydrates,
vitamins, and minerals?**

The biggest advantage to serving fruit juices is that kids
are likely to accept them, which leads to a disadvantage:
They'll drink juice to the exclusion of other foods. (A

child who has consumed three to four glasses of apple juice is not going to be very hungry at dinnertime.) Fruit juices, particularly apple juice, can also cause diarrhea, which can lead to excess fluid loss, which, in turn, can cause vitamin and mineral deficiencies. Unlike whole fruits, juices are not a good source of fiber. All of this does not mean that fruit juices should be avoided. Rather, they should be served in small quantities—no more than 4 to 6 ounces a day—or diluted with water.

As far as cereal is concerned, my kids only like the pre-sweetened kind. Are these okay?

While presweetened cereals are usually loaded with sugar, most are vitamin-fortified, generally to the 25 percent Recommended-Dietary-Allowance level. While a steady diet of highly sweetened cereals is to be avoided, recent research shows that children who begin the day with fortified cereal are far better nourished than those who skip breakfast altogether. They are also somewhat ahead of those who start the day with the traditional, high-fat bacon-and-eggs combo.

Other Foods

What about liquids?

While all foods contain some liquids, we do need to consume liquids separately, too. Plain water is one of our best sources of liquid, though most of us don't drink as much as we should. Children, particularly, rarely choose water to quench their thirsts. Milk, of course, is a desirable liquid food, and young children need the calcium and fat that come from whole milk. Adults and older children can get the calcium they need, without unnecessary fats, by drinking low-fat or nonfat milk. Because it is so good for them, it's easy for parents to encourage children to drink huge quantities of milk. Too much milk, however (more than a quart a day for young children or adults or more than a quart and a half a day for older kids and teens), can lead to low iron levels because excess calcium can block the absorption of iron. A pint a day is really enough for young children and adults, while teens may need as much as a quart. And, like too much fruit juice, too much milk can inhibit the appetite for other foods. Soda pop, a popular drink among many families, is not a good source of nutrition, and the caffeine contained in some soft drinks can be harmful to kids. (For more on the effects of caffeine on young children, see pages 144–145.)

How can I be sure my family is getting enough vitamins and minerals? Should I give them vitamin supplements?

Both children and adults who eat a variety of foods are likely to be getting all the vitamins and minerals they need in their diets and, therefore, don't need any supplemental vitamins. The exceptions are nursing infants and pregnant and nursing women, who should have a vitamin-D supplement added to their diets; and pregnant and nursing women, who need an iron supplement. (Bottle-fed infants should be having vitamin-D-fortified formula.) Children and adults who have been ill and unable or unwilling to eat balanced meals for more than a few days may benefit from a supplement. Before self-prescribing, however, it's a good idea to check with a medical professional.

What about "junk" food? Do we have to give up dessert and snack foods?

Desserts need not be considered "junk food"—especially if you're serving custard, baked apples, or other fruit dishes. The empty-calorie desserts, such as cake or cookies, will do no real harm either, if eaten occasionally and in moderation. It's important that children not learn to view these foods as prizes to be awarded only after the "icky" (in other words, *nutritious)* foods are eaten. This practice teaches kids to overvalue certain sweet foods and to undervalue more nutritious foods.

As far as snack foods are concerned, potato chips, corn chips, and other high-fat, high-salt foods contain little real nutrient value (other than providing calories for energy) and should take up a very small corner of any shopping basket. (It's worth noting that in some families, 25 percent of the weekly grocery bill goes to these nutritionally weak foods.) Good snack foods include fresh or dried fruits; cheese and crackers; peanut butter and all-fruit jam on bread; flavored or plain milk or yogurt; raw vegetables and yogurt dips; nuts and seeds (for older children and adults); and low-salt pretzels.

Helping Your Family to Eat Right

Once the shopping is done, the next step is figuring out how to get these wholesome foods into your family. The most important rule to remember is that even though almost everyone can and should eat the same variety of foods, the quantities and forms in which foods are served will be somewhat different for different family members. Logic

43

doesn't always have much to do with it. For instance, a child of six weighing 50 pounds needs as much iron and calcium, and more vitamin D (for bone growth), than a twenty-five-year-old man. He also needs proportionally more thiamine, riboflavin, niacin, and vitamins A, C, B_6, and B_{12} for his body size than does an adult.

Because children grow in spurts, they need an increased amount of food during rapid-growth periods and somewhat less food for their body weights during slower-growth periods. As they move from babyhood to childhood, however, their overall needs will increase. An average one-year-old consumes about 1,000 calories a day. By age three, he eats about 1,300 calories each day; and by the time he's six, it's up to 1,700 calories. By the early teen years, girls need around 2,200 and boys almost 3,000 calories a day. Individual children, of course, may need fewer or more calories depending on such variables as activity level and basal metabolism rates.

Children's appetites vary a great deal, too, just as adults' do. The same child may have a different level of appetite from one phase of development to the next: He may be a terrific eater at age one and a picky eater at three, for instance. His desire for food can vary from day to day, too, depending on how active he is, what kinds of foods he prefers at the moment, and whether he's feeling well. One possible signal of impending growth is an across-the-board increase in food consumption by a child. The opposite can be true, too. When a child's eating slows down but he seems healthy in all respects, he has probably entered a period of slower growth.

The nutritional needs of children and adults can be best met by serving well-balanced meals and a healthful variety of snacks, of course. But no meal-by-meal checklist is needed. Even a month-long food jag will not undo a child's good health. What counts in the long run is that a child learns to eat a variety of foods in an unstressed atmosphere and that, as he grows, he learns to navigate the social aspects of food and ultimately, learns to choose a nutritionally sound diet for himself.

● ●

Dealing with the Picky Eater

- Don't use food as a pacifier, reward, or punishment. These gimmicks bestow an emotional value to food that can begin a lifelong inappropriate response to eating.

- Don't worry about how *little* your child eats. The average child increases his weight 300 percent in the first year but only 12 percent a year between ages three and five. Less food is required to support this slower rate of growth. If your child's growth is within the normal range, he is eating enough.

- Set a good example. If you eat erratically and make poor food choices, you can expect your child to do the same.

- Limit the amount of less-desirable food kept in the house. Don't however, make any food "off limits." Sweets and treats are fine in moderation.

- If your child doesn't like one category of foods, offer a nutritional equivalent: Substitute fruits for vegetables, replace meat with fish, poultry, cheese, eggs, or peanut butter.

- Have your child select three different foods at each meal. Though the combination may be unusual—meatloaf, a banana, and a slice of bread—it will provide variety, which is one cornerstone of good nutrition.

- Let your child be a "kitchen helper." Let him select foods at the supermarket and help prepare meals. Children who help make foods are more likely to eat them.

- Stay calm and maintain a sense of humor.

Source: From *The Yummy or Yucky Taste Test,* by Jo-Ann Heslin, M.A., R.D., and Annette Natow, Ph.D., R.D. Reprinted from *Sesame Street Parents' Guide,* April 1988.

Feeding and Medicating the Sick Child

Feeding a child during illness can be difficult. Most children lose their appetites when they're not feeling well, and they don't feel like eating much of anything. They often get cranky, too, which makes it doubly difficult when you try to convince them to eat. Try not to worry too much about a child's not eating properly during a brief illness. Most children bounce back quickly from illness and rapidly resume normal eating habits.

All you can do during the sick days is to try to make the child comfortable and provide appealing foods. Consider the symptoms and think about what you might like if you were in your child's shoes. For instance, children with colds often enjoy warm lemonade, soups, and cocoa, just as you do. Children with sore throats that are unrelated to phlegm-producing colds may go for ice-cream, pudding, frozen-pudding pops, and custard. A child with an upset stomach probably won't want anything, but as he begins to feel a little better, toast or a plain cookie might prove tempting.

Many children don't even feel like drinking liquids when they're sick, but it is more important for them to maintain fluid consumption than to eat solid foods. Try to coax your child into drinking something. A child often prefers cold drinks when he runs a fever, hot drinks when a chill is on. Any particular concerns you have about your child's diet during an illness should be discussed with a medical professional.

When you have to give a child medication, there are a few strategies worth remembering that might make a difficult time easier. Young children usually have medicine prescribed in liquid form. For infants up to three months, it's best administered through a nipple. Prop the child up so that he's facing you, perhaps in a baby seat. Place a nipple in the baby's mouth and, using an infant bulb syringe or dropper, drop the medicine (which should be at room temperature) into the nipple and let the baby suck the medicine. If the baby is unable to suck, use the syringe to drop the medication directly into the baby's mouth, toward the back of the mouth or along the gums. You'll have better luck if you give your baby his medicine when he's hungry.

If there are young children in the house who need to take medicine by bulb syringe, *boil* the syringe following each use. Otherwise, germs can be sucked back into the syringe and can prolong the child's illness, negating some of the medication's benefits.

Chilling medicine makes it more palatable to toddlers and preschoolers, who usually take medicine in liquid form from a spoon. For those who balk at taking any ill-tasting liquid medication, you can try mixing the medication in a pleasant-tasting food such as chocolate milk or gelatin. Some medicines are given in tasty, chewable tablets. Children should be told that they are taking medicine, *not* candy. And like all medications, children's medicine should be kept well out of their reach, especially those that are sweet tasting, and thus tempting, to young children.

● ●

CHAPTER FOUR

• • • • • •

How Does the Body Use Food?

Food is the fuel that keeps our bodies running, providing the energy to keep the heart beating, the lungs inflating, the blood circulating, the digestive tract working, and the nerves and muscles operating. The body cannot live without fuel, regardless of whether it's active, at rest, or asleep. Just like a car, the body uses less fuel when it's idling than when it's racing. But food is more than basic fuel. Food also provides the substances needed to replace, repair, and create tissues and protect cells from invaders, such as disease. For children and adolescents, food also plays a dramatic role in physical and mental growth.

The body uses some fuel right away, but it also stores certain substances so that they can be used later, when they're needed. During strenuous physical exertion, for example, the body needs extra energy to fuel the increased activity asked of it. Likewise, during the rapid growth spurts of toddlerhood and adolescence, the body demands more food than at other times. Any excess food that is not needed to fuel additional activity or growth is stored by the body as fat, while too little fuel during a period when it is greatly needed can result in malnutrition.

The process by which our bodies break down the food we eat is known as *digestion*. During digestion, the nutrients in food are changed into forms that can be absorbed and delivered to the hungry cells. Digestion involves a number of mechanical and chemical processes that are variously suited to help retrieve specific nutrients. Mechanical processes, including chewing and the churning of the stomach, act throughout the entire cycle of digestion, as do some chemical processes, which, by means of acids and enzymes, work on the compounds found in the foods we eat. Proteins, carbohydrates, and fats must be broken down for absorption, while vitamins and minerals are absorbed by the body in their original form.

The Incredible Journey

While the digestive process can be triggered by smells, actual digestion begins with the first bite we take—or in the case of toothless infants, with the first drop that reaches the tongue. As we chew solids or as we drink liquids, the saliva in our mouths begins to break down the starches in these foods into molecules of simpler, more easily digestible sugars.

When we swallow, wavelike muscular motions called *peristalsis* carry food down the esophagus and through the cardiac sphincter into the stomach. There, the mechanical and chemical actions continue. The first foods consumed at a meal migrate toward the outer edges of the stomach; foods eaten later go toward the center. The outer portions of the stomach add gastric juices to the mixture. These juices contain hydrochloric acid, which aids in the splitting of proteins and the destruction of harmful microorganisms; mucin, which is a lubricant that protects the digestive tract and helps to move food along in it; and the enzymes pepsin and gastric lipase, which help to split proteins and fat molecules, respectively.

The amount of gastric juice present in the stomach is affected by the way we think and react. It increases with pleasant smells, tastes, and thoughts about food, and it is inhibited by unpleasant odors and sights and by emotions such as fear or anger. There really is truth to the theory that pleasant mealtimes help people digest their food better; conversely, heated arguments at the dinner table really can cause indigestion.

Food remains in the stomach for an average of four hours, although some foods, such as some carbohydrates, can be processed and leave the stomach in as little as thirty minutes. Fats take the longest time to be digested, which is why foods high in fat make us feel fuller longer. Proteins take longer to be digested than carbohydrates but quite a bit less time than fats. The more food of all types that is eaten, the longer it takes the stomach to process its contents; that is why eating meals that contain the right proportions of protein, carbohydrates, and fats keeps us feeling full longer.

Once the stomach's processes are completed, the food is carried into the small intestine.

Some of the most important of the digestive processes take place while food is in the small intestine. At this time, other juices are secreted that help to break down food further, in order to make it available to the system. The pancreas secretes pancreatic juices containing enzymes, which are capable of splitting proteins, carbohydrates, fats, and their subcomponents. The juices also contain bicarbonate, which neutralizes the acid added in the stomach. The liver secretes bile, which helps to digest fats by emulsifying them, thus making them available to the absorptive processes. Last but not least, the cells of the intestinal lining produce a juice that contains enzymes for processing carbohydrates, proteins, and fats.

While the pancreas and liver perform their chemical duties, the food is carried through the small intestine by the rhythmic movement of the intestinal wall. As this happens, the food brushes against the villi, small projections that line the wall of the small intestine at the site of absorption. The villi are so efficient that nearly 95 percent of key nutrients will have been absorbed once the food has passed through the small intestine.

The nutrients extracted by the villi are delivered to the bloodstream in several ways. Vitamins, minerals, and the nutrient molecules of carbohydrates and proteins are absorbed primarily by the blood capillaries. The end products of fats enter the lymphatic ducts and are transported from there into the bloodstream. When the elements reach the cells, via the bloodstream, they will be used for building and repairing tissue and regulating body functions, or they will be stored for later use. Any nutrients not absorbed by the small intestine will be handled by the large intestine.

The large intestine is the final stage along the food's journey. It absorbs excess fluid and dissolves mineral salts to help maintain the body's fluid balance. Extra water is flushed (along with other waste products) through the kidneys. The large intestine also helps in the formation of feces, the body's solid waste. This waste, which is about two-thirds water and one-third solids (fiber, fat, and minerals), also includes large amounts of bacteria and sloughed cells from the small intestine.

The digestive processes work in essentially the same way for everyone, old or young, although newborn babies' systems are not fully developed. (That's one important reason for not feeding solid foods to infants, even if they are capable of eating them.) Within four to six months, however, a baby's system has usually developed to the point at which foods other than breast milk or formula can be tolerated.

Dealing with Indigestion-Related Discomforts

"I can't believe I ate the whole thing" was the refrain of an award-winning advertisement of a generation ago. One of the reasons the ad was so successful was that practically everyone could identify with the poor guy who said it. We've all made ourselves uncomfortable as a result of something we've eaten—or overeaten.

Flatulence

All of us, even babies, experience flatulence—what we usually call *gas*—at one time or another. The feeling is that of being bloated, and it is often accompanied by abdominal cramps. Flatulence is not a particularly serious medical problem, but it can be painful. In infants, this painful cramping is called *colic*.

The most common cause of gas is swallowed air, but certain foods may produce the sensation as well. The foods that most commonly cause gas include carbonated beverages, dried peas and beans, cabbage, broccoli, brussels sprouts, cauliflower, salad greens, fruit, milk, yogurt, and cheese. Some people are particularly sensitive to carrots, raisins, bananas, apricots, prune juice, citrus fruits, apples, pretzels, bagels, bread, pastries, wheat germ, potatoes, or eggplant.

If you or your older child seem to suffer particularly from gas, try eliminating offending foods from your diets to see if the condition improves. Keep in mind that a child's tolerance for various foods is always changing. What gave your child gas last month may be fine for her today.

● ●

Dealing with Colic

Your infant is well fed and for a moment or two after feeding, she seems content. Then she begins kicking and screaming, her whole body moving in spasms. How can you comfort her? While no solution has been found that works for every colicky child, the following tips have worked for many:

- Mothers of breast-fed infants can try to eliminate gas-causing foods from their own diets.

- Parents of bottle-fed babies can try switching from cow-milk–based to soybean-based formulas.

- Infants can be placed on their stomachs, either in a bed or across your legs, and patted vigorously (though not too vigorously).

- Some infants respond well to swaddling.

- Devices such as lambswool pads, bouncing (not rocking) cradles, and vibrating pads help soothe many colicky infants.

- Monotonous, droning sounds accompanied by steady vibration can help, too, and some parents find that placing a colicky infant atop the washer, dryer, or dishwasher has a calming effect. (Just be sure to stay with the infant, as vibrations can cause an infant seat to travel.) A car trip, too, can lull a screaming infant to sleep.

- While knowing that colic never lasts beyond an infant's fourth month may not soothe the child, it can help parents get through the experience.

● ●

Diarrhea

Like gas, diarrhea attacks practically everyone at one time or another. It occurs when food travels too rapidly through the intestines for fluid to be extracted or when the cells lining the intestines add extra water. The result is abdominal cramps and frequent, watery stools.

The possible causes are many: bacterial infections, the ingestion of spoiled food, nervous tension, overeating, and the ingestion of foods and spices that irritate the gastrointestinal tract. Diarrhea usually lasts no longer than twenty-four hours in a child. If it does last longer, consult your pediatrician, as it may be a symptom of a serious illness, and in and of itself, it can cause dehydration which if untreated can be fatal.

Although its causes are many and varied, there are precautions you can take to lessen the chances of diet-produced diarrhea, particularly in children. Some experts suggest that you avoid eating very spicy foods while nursing a baby, as some of the spices can be absorbed into breast milk and cause irritation. Don't feed children highly spiced foods or let them drink too many fruit juices, either. Apple juice, a real favorite with toddlers, often causes diarrhea when it is consumed in too-large quantities. Keeping children away from artificially sweetened foods, such as diet sodas and sugar-free lollipops and gum, can help, too.

Carbonated beverages, in general, speed the reaction of the intestines by causing the muscles to contract more quickly than normal and so should be avoided by a child who has diarrhea. On the other hand, sodas that have gone flat, especially ginger ale, can help to calm the stomach. Anyone experiencing diarrhea should drink plenty of liquids to avoid dehydration. These can include water, weak tea, gelatin mixed with water, ice cubes, or Popsicles.

If your baby has diarrhea and is bottle-fed, you should check with your physician to determine if you can temporarily reduce the strength of her formula. If your baby can take solid food, feed her a little mashed banana or applesauce, both of which contain pectin, which helps firm the stool. The same goes for older children. As a child begins to feel better, give her bland foods, such as toast and rice.

Constipation

On the opposite end of the scale from diarrhea is constipation, characterized by infrequent bowel movements and hard, dry stools. Many parents worry about constipation in their children, but it's helpful to know that everyone's habits are different, and not every child needs a bowel movement every day. More important than the frequency of bowel movements is whether they are difficult to pass. Know what your child's normal routine is so you will be aware if and when it changes.

Constipation is caused by many things, including nervous tension and lack of exercise. The key to preventing constipation is to drink plenty of fluids, to exercise, and to eat a variety of foods, including those high in fiber. (For more on fiber, see page 33.)

A more serious cause of apparent constipation is bowel obstruction, which can be caused if a child accidentally ingests petroleum jelly or other like substances (such as lotions or ointments). If you suspect that bowel obstruction is a possibility, consult your doctor immediately. Whatever the cause of your child's constipation, *never* give her laxatives without first consulting a health professional.

Food Allergies and Sensitivities

Food allergies in children can be particularly worrisome to parents. It's always distressing when the good food we give our kids makes them miserable, whether the reaction is as minor as a few sniffles and a rash or as serious as vomiting and diarrhea.

Food allergies are actually quite rare, though they do tend to run in families. If one parent has an allergy, a child has a 40 percent chance of developing a food sensitivity before the age of twelve. If both parents have allergies, there's a 75 percent chance that a child will develop one or more allergies by age six. Age is a factor, too; the younger the child, the greater her chance of developing a reaction to an allergy-causing substance. There is no way of predicting a child's response to any particular food. The symptoms of an allergy or sensitivity may vary from person to person within a family, too. One person may develop eczema, a form of skin rash, in response to a certain food, while another one may wheeze or develop hives.

Most allergy problems in children develop during infancy. Feeding an infant breast milk has been shown to decrease the likelihood of her developing allergies, but for those who don't breast-feed, simply delaying the introduction of solid food to an infant's diet until she is about six months of age will help greatly. Such foods as wheat, egg whites, cow's milk, soy products, citrus fruits, and seafood can cause allergic reactions in children under the age of one.

How can you tell if a baby or child is sensitive to a particular food? If she develops colic, vomits excessively after eating, has diarrhea, eczema, a runny nose, hives, or wheezing, she may be having a reaction to food. Other, more serious, symptoms such as unexplained weight loss, blood in the stool, or vomiting can also be caused by allergies, but immediate attention to these symptoms is crucial to rule out any more serious condition. The most serious reaction to food is shock, characterized by pale skin, profuse sweating, weak pulse, and, ultimately, unconsciousness. This reaction, though extremely rare, can be fatal if not treated immediately. Medical intervention is essential.

If you suspect that your child is sensitive or truly allergic to a food, consult with your pediatrician or local hospital for the name of a qualified nutritionist or allergist who can help determine the source of the allergy and develop a sound diet for your child.

• •
Dealing with Milk-Product Allergies

Some children and adults have difficulty digesting milk. This is known as *lactose intolerance,* and it develops when sensitive people eat more than a certain amount of milk and milk products. The symptoms include gas, bloating, abdominal cramps, and diarrhea.

For the lactose in milk to be used by the body, it must be broken down into its component sugars, glucose and galactose, by the enzyme lactase, found in the intestinal tract. Lactase levels are high at birth and through the first year or two of life for almost all humans, which is why milk intolerance is rare in infants. After that, lactase diminishes, and in some people it disappears.

Tolerance to milk varies from person to person. For most people with lactose intolerance, the problem develops gradually. A typical sufferer is still able to drink some quantity of milk as she grows older, but amounts that were once easily digested begin to cause discomfort. Over time, the intolerance increases, and the amount of milk products consumed must be reduced.

Lactose is found in all dairy products, but that doesn't mean that people who are lactose-intolerant must resign themselves to a life without milk. There are alternatives. For those who cannot eat milk itself, cultured milk products such as ripened cheese, yogurt, buttermilk, and sour cream are good alternatives. Many lactose-intolerant people drink sweet acidophilus milk, which tastes just like ordinary milk but is much easier to digest, thanks to the addition of acidophilus bacteria in the processing. Others add lactase tablets to regular milk. This changes the taste of the milk slightly, however, making it a little sweeter. Those who are unable to tolerate milk can also use soybean-based milk substitutes. Calcium needs can be met by eating sardines, canned salmon, and calcium-fortified orange juice. (See pages 29–30 for a more complete listing of high-calcium foods.)

• •

PART II
......
The Nutritional Needs of Children

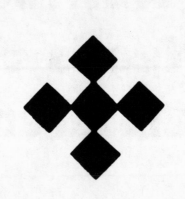

Introduction to Part II

● ● ● ● ● ●

"You're *not* breast-feeding?!!"

—from a well-meaning in-law

"That's yucky!"

—from your toddler

"I'm not hungry."

—from your eight-year-old

"I already ate."

—from your preteen

"Meat loaf again! I'm going out for pizza."

—from your almost-grown teen

This litany of food-related exclamations is familiar in any household. What's a parent to do? We all want to feed our kids right, but what kids will eat is not always what we'd like them to eat. We'd like to start this section by assuring you that your child is not the only one who seems to subsist on peanut butter and jelly sandwiches. Nor are you the only parent who worries if your kids are eating enough or well enough. It helps to know, too, that most children will respond to your concern that they eat nutritiously once they understand that eating well doesn't necessarily mean eating things they don't like.

In this section, we'll discuss the specific dietary needs of children at various ages and some of the kid-pleasing foods that can provide these needs. We also include a special section on eating disorders.

CHAPTER FIVE

······

The Nutritional Needs of Infants

When you get up in the middle of the night to breast-feed your child or give her a warm bottle, and you're sitting in the rocker, bleary-eyed from lack of sleep, you may find it hard to believe that feeding a child during her first year of life is as easy as it will ever get, at least as far as food choices are concerned. Granted, her timing may not be perfect, but an infant's needs are simple.

For the first few months, a baby requires only breast milk and perhaps a vitamin D supplement or an iron-fortified formula. Between the ages of four to six months, most children are ready to be introduced to solid foods, often beginning with such soft foods as a single-grain cereal and applesauce and moving on to other pureed selections. By the end of the first year, she has also completed the most intense period of growth she will ever experience, often tripling her birth weight. By this time, she's usually coping with scrambled eggs, cottage cheese, and other adult foods like a real pro.

How Much Food Do Babies Need?

Because of her rapid growth, a baby's food needs, while simple, are fairly constant. Newborns generally eat 2 to 3 ounces of food every two to four hours. After three or four months, most babies need to eat less frequently, but they eat greater amounts—usually five or six times a day and about 5 or 6 ounces at a time, for a total of about 30 to 32 ounces a day. Naturally, consumption varies from baby to baby.

Infants generally eat until they are satisfied, and letting them start and stop when they wish is a good way to ensure that they're getting as much food as they need. If they become uncomfortable, crying and possibly spitting up often during a feeding, they may be indicating that they've had more than enough. Overfeeding typically occurs with bottle-fed babies, usually because they're encouraged to finish their bottles even when they're full. When babies are breast-fed, there is no bottle to finish and, the babies themselves are more likely to determine that mealtime is over.

Babies can be underfed as well. When an infant drinks a whole bottle and still seems upset, it may be because she's still hungry. Breast-fed infants can eat too little, too, if the breast is removed before they've had enough. Since you can't determine how much is being consumed, it can be hard to know. The best gauge is the baby's rate of growth.

How do you know if your baby is growing properly? If she seems contented most of the time and is getting noticeably bigger, you can be fairly sure that she is getting proper nourishment. It's helpful to know that a baby who wets a minimum of six diapers per day is probably eating plenty. If you're unsure, weigh your baby every week or two. Most infants gain 6 to 8 ounces a week and grow about an inch per month for the first three months. For the next three months, the length growth continues at about three quarters of an inch a month, but the weight gain slows to about 5 or 6 ounces a week. For the next six months, they average 2 or 3 ounces each week and grow about half an inch each month. It's important to remember that no two babies follow the same growth pattern and that there is, within the normal range, a great variety, as the graphs on pages 67–70 show.

GIRLS FROM BIRTH TO 36 MONTHS
WEIGHT FOR AGE

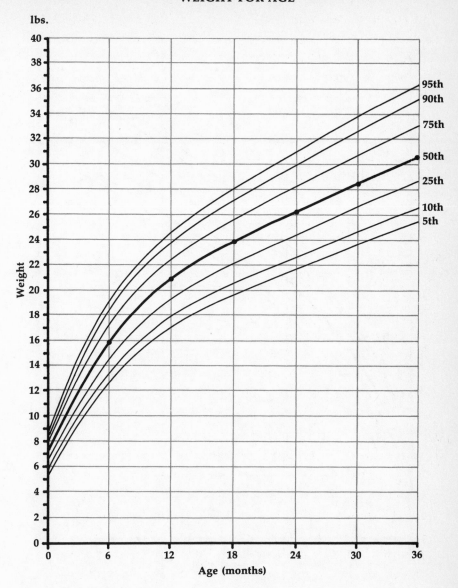

Source: Department of Health, Education and Welfare, Public Health Service, Health Resources Administration, National Center for Health Statistics, and Center for Disease Control.

GIRLS FROM BIRTH TO 36 MONTHS
LENGTH FOR AGE

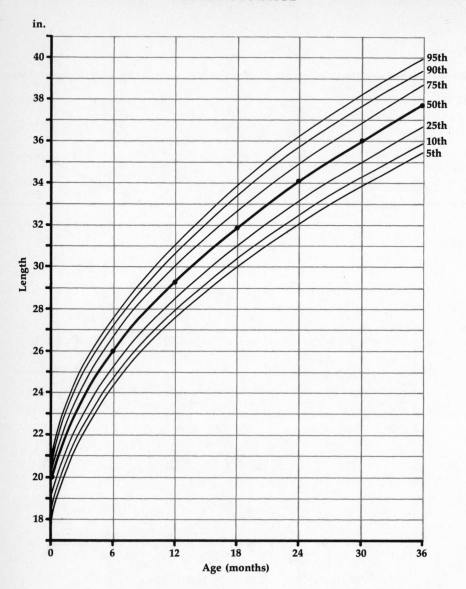

in.

Length

Age (months)

95th
90th
75th
50th
25th
10th
5th

Source: Department of Health, Education and Welfare, Public Health Service, Health Resources Administration, National Center for Health Statistics, and Center for Disease Control.

BOYS FROM BIRTH TO 36 MONTHS
WEIGHT FOR AGE

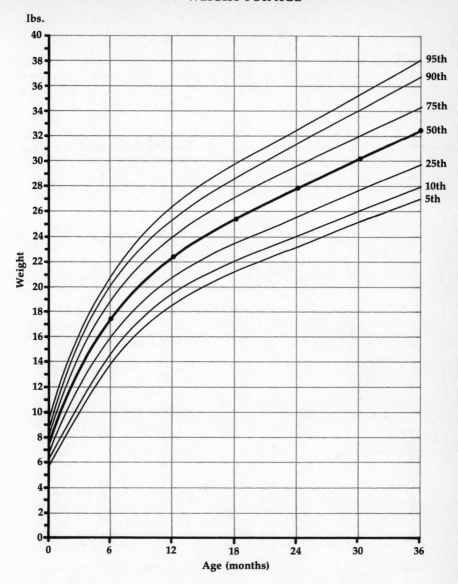

Source: Department of Health, Education and Welfare, Public Health Service, Health Resources Administration, National Center for Health Statistics, and Center for Disease Control.

BOYS FROM BIRTH TO 36 MONTHS
LENGTH FOR AGE

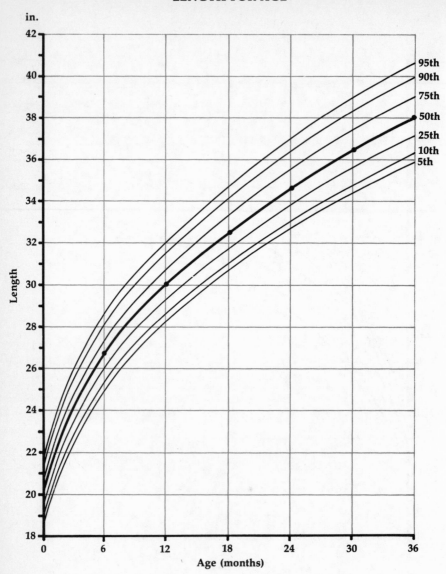

Source: Department of Health, Education and Welfare, Public Health Service, Health Resources Administration, National Center for Health Statistics, and Center for Disease Control.

• •

All About Growth Charts

A standard part of most visits to the pediatrician is reviewing the growth chart. Your doctor will plot your child's weight for age, length or height for age, and weight for length at regular intervals. You should ask your doctor to take some time to explain the growth chart to you.

Growth charts are based on weight and height measurements of thousands of American children. The results are given as *percentiles.* Your doctor may tell you, for example, that your child is at the fiftieth percentile for height, the twenty-fifth percentile for weight, and somewhere between the twenty-fifth and fiftieth percentiles for weight for length. This means that, compared to other girls her age, she is about average for height, a little less than average for weight, and that her weight for her length is also just a little less than average. Children may measure in the average range, below average, or even well above average and still be perfectly normal and healthy. What is most important is how *steadily* the child grows over time.

Growth is affected by heredity, health status, and, of course, nutrition. A child may stop growing temporarily during an illness or infection. She will usually make up this growth when she is well again, as long as her diet is good. This is called *catch-up growth.*

Children also experience growth spurts during which they will grow very rapidly over the course of a few weeks, months, or, during adolescence, years. (Iron-deficiency anemia is a common side effect of rapid growth, and all children should be closely monitored for this.) On average, boys are slightly longer and heavier than girls from birth through childhood. Since girls generally reach puberty about two years sooner than boys, there will be a period of time, usually between ages nine and fourteen, when girls will be taller and heavier than boys. Female hormones hasten the closure of the growth ends of bones, and most girls will have attained their adult heights by age fourteen or fifteen. Boys continue to grow until age eighteen or even beyond.

Growth can also affect different parts of the body at different times. Children are quite sensitive about this and do not appreciate jokes about how their feet arrive in a room several minutes before the rest of them. Many children, especially the late and early bloomers, have a lot of concerns about their size. A sensitive pediatrician or guidance counselor can be very helpful in allaying their anxieties. Since it is natural for many children to put on some extra fat just before their adolescent growth spurt, parents should be cautious before jumping to the conclusion that the child is becoming obese. In addition, girls add fat layers during puberty. These fat layers provide a caloric reserve for later childbearing and give the female her characteristic shape. Jokes about this process from friends and relatives can lay the foundation for eating disorders in an already sensitive child.

On page 73 is a list of *average* weights and heights (the fiftieth percentile) for both boys and girls at various ages. Remember, however, that there is a great deal of variation from child to child. Also, growth charts were standardized on white, middle-class children. Children of different ethnic backgrounds may vary markedly from these norms.

Average Heights and Weights

| | Girls | | | Boys | |
Age	Height	Weight	Age	Height	Weight
2	34"	26 lbs	2	34"	27 lbs
3	37"	31.5 lbs	3	37.5"	32 lbs
4	40"	36 lbs	4	41.5"	36.5 lbs
5	43"	39 lbs	5	43.5"	41 lbs
6	45"	43 lbs	6	46"	46 lbs
9	52"	62.5 lbs	9	52"	62 lbs
10	54.5"	72 lbs	10	54"	70 lbs
12	60"	92 lbs	12	59"	88 lbs
14	63"	110 lbs	14	64"	112 lbs
18	64.5"	125 lbs	18	69.5"	152 lbs

Source: Kathleen Carpenter, M.S., R.D.

• •

To Breast-Feed or Bottle-Feed?

The choice as to whether or not to breast-feed is a highly personal one. And for some mothers, matters of personal comfort, medical considerations, and the ability to produce milk limit the choice to bottle-feeding. Parents who opt for bottle-feeding can be assured that they are not nutritionally shortchanging their baby, since today's formulas do well in mimicking the nutritional content of mother's milk. Most infant formulas are based on modified cow's milk or soy proteins, have a high carbohydrate content, a balance of needed vitamins and minerals, and are easy to digest. Bottle-feeding has the advantage of allowing fathers to participate equally in their baby's feedings.

Breast-feeding has distinct advantages, however, the primary one being that mother's milk contains antibodies that give the infant some immunity to diseases until her own immune system develops, at about six months of age. Recent research even suggests that breast milk may contain substances that stimulate, or "turn on," the infant's immune system. Studies show that breast-fed babies are also less likely to develop food allergies later in life, since foods likely to cause problems are introduced after the baby's system has developed to a point at which it is less easily irritated.

Breast-feeding generally requires little extra equipment and is convenient in that there is no formula to mix, nothing to heat or cool, and no bottles to wash. (Breast pumps and bottles are needed, of course, for mothers who must be away during some of their baby's mealtimes.)

As far as "bonding" is concerned, both breast-feeding and bottle-feeding allow parents to make the necessary intimate connection with their newborns. All that's required is that feeding time be a time of loving touch, eye contact, and comfort.

....

CONSUMER TIP: Microwave ovens are a boon to busy parents, but baby bottles should *never* be heated in them. There's always a possibility that some portion of the milk or formula has reached the scalding point.

....

• •

Daily Food Guide for Nursing Mothers

Food Group	Servings Needed	One Serving Is:
Milk and milk products	4–5	1 cup milk 1⅓ cups cottage cheese 1½ oz cheese 1½ cups ice cream 1 cup yogurt

Protein foods
  animal (2 servings)
  vegetable (2 servings)
	4 or more	1 egg
		1 oz cooked meat, fish, or poultry
		½ cup cooked beans
		2 tbsp peanut butter
		1 oz nuts or seeds

Breads and cereals	4 or more	1 slice bread ½ cup hot cereal, cooked ¾ cup cold cereal ½ cup rice, noodles, pasta 1 tortilla
Dark green and dark yellow vegetables	1	¾ cup raw ½ cup cooked
Vitamin C-rich fruits and vegetables	2	½ cup raw ¾ cup cooked

Food Group	Servings Needed	One Serving Is:
Vitamin C-rich fruits and vegetables (continued)	2	$1/2$ cup orange/ grapefruit juice 1 medium fruit or vegetable
Other fruits and vegetables	1 or more	$3/4$ cup raw $1/2$ cup cooked 1 medium fruit or vegetable

• •

Vitamin and Mineral Supplements

Babies who are fed formula don't usually need vitamin and mineral supplements, since formulas are fortified with all the needed nutrients, especially iron-fortified formulas. Breast-fed babies are usually given vitamin-D supplements, since mother's milk contains relatively little vitamin D. While they're still in the womb, babies take on stores of iron from their mothers, but by about three months of age, those iron stores become depleted. It is a good idea to use iron-fortified formula from birth onward. Despite what you might have heard, the iron-fortified formulas are not associated with any greater incidence of digestive upset than low-iron formulas. Since breast milk provides little iron, breast-fed babies are sometimes given iron supplements as a preventive measure, to be replaced with an iron-fortified cereal once solid foods are introduced. Iron supplements, like any other supplements, should be given to a baby only on the instructions of a medical professional.

Getting Them Started on Solid Foods

In the past, parents were told they could start their babies on solid foods almost as soon as they were home—anywhere from a few days to two weeks old. Today, however, most parents are encouraged to keep babies on breast milk or formula exclusively until their babies' digestive systems are more developed. The reason for this change in timing is that babies have been found to develop fewer allergic reactions to foods after the age of four to six months.

How do you know when your baby is ready for solid food? Technically, babies are ready to add solid foods to their diets when they are able to transfer food from the front of their mouth to the back for swallowing. How do you know when this has happened? All babies have a sucking reflex, during which they usually stick their tongues out. At a certain point, usually during or after the fourth month, babies become less interested in sucking. You will be able to tell when your baby is ready for food when her tongue no longer appears automatically when something is placed in her mouth. When you begin introducing solid foods, serve them on a spoon, never mixed in with bottled formula. This allows your baby to exercise her mouth muscles.

The other change that makes spoon-feeding possible is the baby's development of head and trunk control. When your baby is able to sit in a high chair or baby seat and lean forward with an open mouth, it is much easier for her to eat than when she was lying down at a 45-degree angle. If you try to feed an infant solid foods before she is able to hold up her head and neck, and thus be in a position to reject food, spoon-feeding may well become force-feeding.

Perhaps most important, babies will tell you when they

are ready for solid food. If your baby's eating habits change—if she wakes up in the night hungry when she had previously slept through; or seems to demand more frequent feedings; or still seems hungry after thirty minutes of breast-feeding or an 8-ounce bottle—she's probably ready for solid food. Another signal is a baby who constantly reaches out to grab and chew on everything in sight.

The purpose of introducing foods at four to six months is not really to provide adequate nutrition, for the baby's needs can still be met quite well with formula or breast milk. It's more a matter of giving the baby a chance to explore textures, tastes, and aromas and, as stated earlier, to allow her to practice using the muscles in her mouth.

Babies tend to be intolerant of new foods when they are extremely hungry, so when you're starting to spoon-feed your baby, it's a good idea to give her a partial feeding of whatever's she's used to—breast milk or formula—before trying to introduce the new solid foods. You can start slowly, feeding only a teaspoon or two on a warm spoon, and work up gradually to larger feedings. Solid foods should not replace breast milk or formula entirely during this transition period. Introduce one new food at a time and stay with it for several days. This allows the child to get used to new foods, and it gives you time to see whether she'll have a negative reaction to a given food. If your child develops an allergic reaction, such as a sore bottom, wheezing, vomiting, diarrhea, or a skin rash, discontinue the offending food for a time. By adding foods gradually—one new food every four days, for instance—to the diet, you can tell more easily which foods, if any, are causing problems.

What to Feed

There are no real rules about which specific solid food is best for a baby who is just learning the ropes. Most parents start with rice cereal, followed by fruits and vegetables, finger foods such as toast and crackers, eggs, and finally meats, but the order is in no way compulsory. Infants have definite preferences in food, so you may have to try a few things to see what your baby likes best.

When you *do* begin to give your baby cereals, keep in mind that rice cereals tend to cause fewer allergic reactions in babies than some of the others. Wheat and corn cereals are usually added after about a year, as they may cause allergic reactions in some young babies. No matter what cereal you use, it can be made more appealing to your baby if you mix it with milk, breast milk, or formula as well as water. Remember to spoon-feed rather than bottle-feed. Feeding solids from a bottle keeps an infant from learning how to use her muscles for chewing; these by the way, are the same muscles she needs to develop for speech later on.

CONSUMER TIP: When buying prepared baby foods in jars, buy the one-food variety, such as strained peas or liver, rather than stews and other mixed-food varieties, since the single-food variety is a better nutritional value.

Fruit-fanciers often start their babies on mashed bananas, applesauce, or pureed apricots, pears, peaches, or plums. Some experts say that citrus fruits should be saved until after the first year, since they may cause an allergic reaction (usually diaper rash) in younger babies.

Many parents wonder if they need to serve special, commercially prepared baby foods. For instance, is baby cereal a must, or will the vitamin-fortified cream of rice that you have every morning do just as well? The simple answer is that the choice is up to you.

Many people like to use commercial baby foods because they are nutritious, convenient to prepare, and easy to carry around. However, baby cereals and baby foods in general are heavily processed; their finer texture may be less pleasing to some children than that of your cereal. Pureed table food is just fine, although some of what adults eat may be too highly seasoned for a six-month-old's palate. Babies tend to like food that has the consistency of thickened cream, so you may want to add a little water, milk, or formula to the pureed adult food.

Hold the Honey

While the introduction of most foods relates to taste and texture and is largely a subjective matter, there is one food to avoid—honey. Despite the temptation to flavor foods with honey, don't give it in any form to a child under one year old, as it may contain spores of *Clostridium botulinum*, which can cause a form of botulism in an infant. These spores cause no problem in the older child or adult, as they are rendered harmless by stomach acid. However, the spores may begin to form toxins in the low-acid atmosphere of a baby's stomach. Botulism, a form of food poisoning that can be fatal at any age, is especially dangerous in infants. After the first year, a baby's digestive tract is able to destroy the spores in honey, so you can feel free to serve it. Other sweeteners, while unnecessary, are not harmful.

Developing Eating Skills

It's a real thrill, no question about it: One minute your one-year-old is lying in your arms drinking from your breast or from a bottle. The next minute she's sitting up in a baby chair, eating from a spoon, and you're wiping strained prunes off your floor. Not only is your child expanding her repertoire of favorite foods; during this time she's learning some vitally important eating skills.

Finger Foods

At around six to eight months of age, teeth usually begin to appear, and soon after that, children begin to develop control of their thumbs and forefingers. Thus, by the age of nine months, they are adept at the pincer grasp, which is particularly useful in learning the first steps of self-feeding. By this point, babies should have food to chew on and to hold.

Popular foods for finger-feeding include toast, bagels, and crackers. Cooled cooked carrots, cheese, and Cheerios (a perennial favorite among babies) are often popular, too, since they can be grasped easily. Some enjoy hard-cooked, poached, or fried egg yolk, but you might want to avoid egg whites for the first year because they often can bring on an allergic reaction. Other favorites include ground meat, cooked pasta, cooked and cooled vegetables, and bananas. (Save raw vegetables and hard-to-bite fruits for later, to avoid choking hazards.)

By the end of the first year, babies have usually developed molars, which means that they're ready for some heavy-duty chewing. Babies' hand skills are also usually developed enough after twelve to fifteen months to enable them to feed themselves more easily. It is at this point that they can graduate to eating regular table food that has been cut into very small, easy-to-swallow pieces.

Drinking from a Cup

Drinking from a cup is a major advance in a baby's motor-skills development, and most babies are ready to start by about eight or nine months of age. You'll know it's time to introduce the cup when your baby can hold other objects such as bottles or toys fairly well. If you think she's about ready for the big time, let her play with an empty cup for a while, so that she can become familiar with the way it feels. Play a drinking game with her, pretending to sip so that she'll get the general idea of what she's meant to do. After a while, you can put a teaspoon or two of water, fruit juice, milk, or cooled broth into the cup and let her experiment with it. (Keep a sponge or a roll of paper towels handy!) Gradually, as your baby's agility increases, you can add more liquid.

The cup you use can be anything from a specially designed weighted cup with a lid to a weighted cup without a lid to any unweighted, unbreakable cup. If you use a lidless variety, expect your baby to discover the art and science of bubble-blowing. Don't let the behavior worry you. Bubble-blowing is a good way to develop oral muscle control. There will be plenty of time to develop good table manners later on. (For more on manners, see chapter 12.)

● ●

Tips for Making Your Own Baby Food

Making your own baby food is certainly less costly than buy-ing commercially prepared foods, and the process needn't be very time consuming. A food mill or blender will make the job easier, but you can also do fine with some foods just using a fork.

What to Make: Fruits and vegetables are good foods to start with. For older babies, pureed meat and poultry are good, too.

How to Prepare Food:

● Wash, peel, and remove seeds from all fruits. Wash all vegetables.

● Slice or dice. Then bake, boil, or steam until tender.

● Use a food mill, blender, or fork to puree fruit or vegetables. A blender works best for pureeing well-cooked meats.

● Add water, milk, formula, or juice to reach desired consistency. (Babies of four to six months need thinner foods than older babies do.)

● Avoid using any spices, including salt, pepper, and sugar.

How to Store Food:

- Cooked fruits and vegetables can be stored in tightly covered jars in the refrigerator for up to three days. Raw fruits or cooked meats can be stored in the refrigerator for a maximum of two days.

- To store food in the freezer, where it will remain fresh for up to one month, try using ice-cube trays. Fill each cube with food, cover the tray with wax paper, and freeze until the food is solid.

- Once frozen solid, remove the cubes from the tray and place them in a plastic bag. Seal the bag, label it, and date it. Dispose of any unused portions one month from this date.

- To serve frozen food, thaw the cube in the refrigerator, not at room temperature.

- After the cube has thawed, heat until warm (not hot) in a double boiler or in the oven.

- Dispose of any unused thawed portions. *Do not refreeze.*

Source: Division of Nutritional Sciences, New York State College of Human Ecology and New York State College of Agriculture and Life Sciences, Cornell University, Ithaca, NY, and the U.S. Department of Agriculture.

● ●

CHAPTER SIX

· · · · · ·

The Nutritional Needs of Toddlers

The word *toddler* conjures up an image of the cutest, sweetest little creature imaginable trying to make his way across the room without falling down. It doesn't sound at all like the tight-lipped (or screaming) table companion who categorically refuses to eat his lunch.

One of the biggest surprises parents can receive comes when their baby turns into a toddler. After being a voracious eater, he may suddenly become picky and uninterested in food. But the toddler's suddenly decreased appetite reflects only a decreased need for food for the time being. After the first year of intense growth, during which he may have tripled his weight, he is entering a stage during which he'll probably gain only a few ounces a month—between 3 and 7 pounds between his first and second birthdays. Unlike the period of infancy, he is now concerned primarily with things other than food.

Up and moving around, he has become intensely interested in exploring the world around him. And with his new sense of independence, he is less likely to want to sit down to a supper of strained spinach. Once he *does* sit down, he's probably going to be more interested in handling his food than in eating it. It's easy to worry if he's getting enough to eat—and reassuring to know that if he seems healthy and energetic and is growing at a reasonable rate, then he probably is.

The charts in chapter 5 will give you a rough idea of how long and heavy your toddler can be expected to be between the ages of twelve and thirty-six months and approximately how much growth you can expect. As you can see, there is a great variation within the normal range.

Making an issue of eating "enough" may be tempting when you're trying to feed a two-year-old, but it could also set the stage for making mealtime a time to test one another's wills, and that's a habit that could last beyond this temporary too-busy-to-eat stage. To help remove the temptation to measure each mouthful, you can try feeding your toddler at a different time of day if your regular mealtime is a high-energy point for him. Or you can let him leave the table after a few bites to pursue whatever interests him, allowing him to finish eating when he's ready. Giving in to his natural timetable does not mean that you are spoiling your child. It simply means that you're responding to your toddler's present need to explore, which is now greater than his need to learn to sit still—or even to eat a well-balanced meal.

What to Serve

Babies begin to develop teeth during infancy, but it's not until toddlerhood, when a full set of teeth grows in, that a child really begins to use them. At about one year of age, children often have a set of molars, allowing them to chew and even grind some foods.

While a toddler needs soft and moist food to accommodate his limited chewing abilities, particularly in the beginning, he does not need to be fed special food. He can eat the same food as the rest of the family, as long as it is already soft and moist or it can be easily softened and moistened by mashing, pureeing, or straining and adding water, juice, or milk. Many parents consider noodles the perfect food for a toddler, since noodles are easy to prepare, easy and fun to eat, and kids usually love them. Meats will need to be cut into very small pieces to accommodate developing teeth and chewing skills. Young children often like soup but find it difficult to manage, since spooning liquid from a bowl takes more dexterity than spooning solid foods. You can help your child by straining the solids from his soup, putting them into a bowl for spoon-feeding, and pouring the liquid into a cup to be drunk.

You can also choose to serve a young toddler commercial "junior" foods. As with infant foods, packaged foods for the slightly older child are generally nutritious and very convenient. Sometimes a child's eating schedule does not match an adult's, and it can be much easier to open a jar of food than to prepare something special. Commercial foods are expensive, however, and not nutritionally superior to the ones you whip up at home in your blender or food processor. And, as with infant food, look for single-food jars rather than mixed foods, as these tend to be more nutritious. Some parents compromise by taking prepared food on trips, to make feeding easier, and using the home-made foods at home.

A toddler will often have odd food preferences—even more so than he did in late infancy. (For a discussion of common food quirks, see pages 95–97.)

There is no one food that toddlers need more than others. They need a balance of various foods, as all people do, and that balance can come from a number of sources. For instance, milk provides a good combination of protein, carbohydrates, fat, vitamins, calcium, and other minerals. But these nutrients can be found in other dairy products as well, such as yogurt, cottage cheese, ice cream, and pudding. In the same way, an egg can be fixed in any number of ways, and it's just as nutritious in a custard as it is when it's scrambled. Just as a toddler has different tastes and will not appreciate the same books or music as you, his food preferences are likely to be less sophisticated than your own.

Vitamin and Mineral Supplements

The seemingly strange eating habits of toddlers often bring up the question of whether or not you should give them daily vitamins. The short answer is probably not.

Certain vitamins—A, D, E, and K—are fat-soluble and thus may be stored in the body for some time. Those vitamins that are water-soluble, the B vitamins and C, can't be stored for very long and thus must be replenished regularly. All of these vitamins are found in a number of foods, and since your toddler doesn't need great amounts of any of them, you probably don't need to worry about his getting enough. Unless your child has eaten one thing exclusively for more than a week or so, you won't need to bother about multivitamin supplements. Toddler's preferences change quickly enough. They have usually moved on to new foods long before there's any need to worry about vitamin deficiencies.

Iron and calcium are two minerals that you might want to be aware of, however. Iron is found in red meats, beans baked with molasses, prunes, egg yolks, fortified cereals, and leafy green vegetables. (See pages 31–32 for a more extensive list of iron-rich foods.) For toddlers who don't care for meat or eggs, an easy method to ensure that they get enough iron is to continue to offer them iron-fortified cereals. If your child eats adequate amounts of a variety of foods or eats iron-fortified cereals, there's probably no need for an iron supplement.

Calcium is important for toddlers' growing bones and teeth. Making sure your child gets enough calcium isn't usually a problem for those who drink milk or milk-based products. For those who do not or cannot eat milk-based foods, calcium-fortified fruit drinks and cereals or canned fish can provide the necessary calcium. (See pages 29–30 for a more extensive list of calcium-rich foods.)

Self-Feeding Skills

Remember how hard it was the first time you tried to drink from a cup or serve yourself with a spoon or fork? No? Then how about the first time you used chopsticks or tried to walk a few feet on skis or use a word processor? All of these new skills took time to master, the same kind of practice time your toddler will need to master his silverware.

There is nothing much you can do about the natural evolution of a toddler's motor skills, nor should you try; however, there are a few things you can do to keep the chaos down to a minimum and perhaps make the learning process a little easier. First, a lidded cup is useful in the beginning, since a young toddler's ability to steady and guide the cup to his mouth is still developing. By the age of two, most children are pretty adept at reaching their mouths successfully, but many a cup will still be dropped, tipped, and poured over the next few years.

While learning to use a spoon by himself is not essential to good nutrition, it *is* an important beginning to learning the social aspects of eating. It also presents a terrific opportunity for a toddler to experience a self-esteem–building sense of accomplishment. At first, the child will have great difficulty scooping food onto the spoon and guiding it into his mouth. But after just a few months, his wrist will be developed enough to allow him to perfect the scooping and twisting motions. By the age of two, the coordination of wrist and elbow will have advanced to the point where spoon-feeding will essentially be mastered. Then he's ready to begin managing the spearing movement needed to use a fork.

Until that time, however, feeding will be messy, and he will often resort to eating with his hands, which is educational in itself, since handling food to learn its texture, smelling it, and just seeing what it can do is very important for a child. It's all a part of learning about the world around him.

Feeding Techniques

If your toddler is suspicious of new foods, try offering them at the beginning of a meal, when he is hungriest. (This strategy doesn't work with infants; they get impatient when they're hungry.) Place a little of the new food on the plate— a tablespoon or two at a time is plenty—wait two or three minutes, and then place other, well-liked foods on the plate. If your child refuses the new food, don't make a fuss. Wait a few days and try offering it again. His tastes or attitudes may have changed by then.

Toddlers also have a keen sense of fun, a sense that extends, not surprisingly, to food. They love to dunk raw vegetables and fruits into dips made from yogurt, ricotta cheese, cottage cheese, or peanut butter. Piles of shredded vegetables are great fun to play with and, incidentally, to eat. They also like sandwiches cut into funny shapes with cookie cutters. Keeping some of these strategies in mind can help when you're about to introduce a new food to a child who isn't always receptive to experimenting.

One thing that you might want to be aware of in teaching your child about food is that he doesn't have a preconceived notion of the way a meal should be eaten. He doesn't know about first courses and entrees yet. To him, dessert is just as good served at the beginning of a meal as at the end, maybe better. Some parents find that it serves to lessen meal tension later on if dessert is not regarded as a bribe to finish a meal but rather as a natural part of it. If you serve a nutritious dessert, such as fruit salad or custard, there is no reason why it can't be eaten before or along with the rest of the meal.

When to Feed

The concept of "grazing," eating small amounts of food several times a day instead of three big meals, has become popular with adults. It has been all the rage among toddlers for a long, long time. Most small children need five or six small meals a day, or three larger ones supplemented with snacks. Schedule meals and snacks so that your child learns to get hungry, rather than feeling full all the time. Nibbling constantly all day can lead to two problems: First, children will get into the habit of eating when they're not at all hungry, which can create weight problems later on; second, kids who aren't hungry are less inclined to try new foods. Don't prolong hunger, however. Scheduling dinner at six o'clock may suit the rest of the family but this may be a time when a toddler is too tired to eat. A child who is too hungry is no fun whatsoever as a dinner companion. If your child does get too hungry to wait for mealtime, feed him early and then have him sit at the table for a little while to have a snack and simply to socialize with the family. The lesson that the dinner table is a pleasant place to be will serve him well during the next stage of development—when he enters his preschool years.

• •
The Daily Food Needs of Toddlers

Milk and Milk Products:	Four to six ½-cup servings
Meat, Fish, Poultry, and Other High-Protein Foods:	Two to three 1-ounce servings
Fruits and Vegetables:	Four or more servings, including one rich in vitamin C and one rich in vitamin A

- One serving of vegetables is 2 to 3 tablespoons.
- One serving of fruit is about ¼ cup cooked or canned fruit or ½ of a small fresh fruit, such as an apple.

Breads, Cereals, and Pasta:

Three to four servings

- One serving of bread is ½ slice.
- One serving of cooked cereal, rice, or pasta is ¼ cup.
- One serving of dry cereal is ⅓ to ½ cup.

Source: *No-Nonsense Nutrition for Kids,* by Annette B. Natow and Jo-Ann Heslin, copyright ©, 1984. Published by McGraw-Hill, Inc. Used with permission of authors.

• •

A Natural Preference for Sweets

It comes as no surprise to most parents that children love sweets. Even in the womb, an unborn child sucks more vigorously when exposed to a sweetened solution. From the moment of birth, sweet tastes provoke a smile or a pleasant gurgle; sour and bitter tastes, on the other hand, are most often—and most adamantly—rejected. Experts feel that a child's preference for sweets is the result of evolution: When humans selected food by scavenging for edible plants, they learned that parts of plants that were sweet were generally safe. Bitter and sour plants were more often unripe or poisonous. This evolutionary selection process gave humans a keen perception for bitterness—and a natural preference for sweets.

Since the underlying taste of many green vegetables is bitterness, many children grimace at their first taste of strained spinach or other greens. Studies have also shown that individual children are genetically predisposed to a sensitivity to bitterness. Dark green vegetables, for example, may truly taste "yucky" to some children and will be refused—no matter how much parents try to browbeat kids into eating them. Must parents, then, abandon their efforts to provide good nutrition until

93

their child is ready to accept a side dish of spinach? Not at all. But instead of insisting that their children eat what is put on their plates, parents can offer fruits, which are nutritionally equivalent substitutes, instead of vegetables. Peaches as a side dish with pork chops or baked apples alongside meat loaf, for example, are kid-pleasing combinations that won't be rejected.

While waiting for a child's eating preferences to expand, it's important that adults refrain from setting up situations that make any particular foods take on too much importance. The child who defines vegetables as "the things you eat to get ice cream" has learned to devalue an entire category of food that he's been bribed to eat. Often, children will reject these foods well into adulthood once they've learned to associate the foods with mealtime power struggles. Similarly, children learn to overvalue foods that are off-limits or that are used as rewards. To remove unnecessary negative or positive associations from food, parents can instead emphasize variety in their child's menu rather than labeling foods as "good foods" or "bad foods." Parents can also be assured that there are sound psychological and physical benefits to eating the so-called bad foods. Sweet, high-calorie snacks not only add to the pleasure of eating but provide a concentrated source of energy that rapidly growing, active youngsters *need*. Too often, parents may withhold these high-energy foods because they are afraid of causing obesity or future health problems. This is not to say that parents should abandon their roles as snack supervisors. It just means that any food, eaten in moderation, is an acceptable treat.

Source: From *The Yummy or Yucky Taste Test,* by Jo-Ann Heslin, M.A., R.D. and Annette Natow, Ph.D., R.D. Reprinted from *Sesame Street Magazine Parents' Guide,* April 1988.

● ●

• •

Common Food Quirks

One day, your two-year-old happily eats spaghetti. The next day, he wrinkles his nose and clamps his mouth shut. "But you love spaghetti," you say. Yes, he did—yesterday! This sudden about-face actually has very little to do with food. Your toddler is just using the table as the stage for asserting his independence from you. The same holds true for a young child's table manners. Food is not the issue here. The eating process is just one more way to learn about the world. Peas squish and feel mushy when you squeeze them; linguini wiggles off the plate and onto the floor; crackers break into delightful mounds of crumbs. These textural experiences, though messy, are very educational. Asking a child to help prepare a meal lets the child experiment in a positive, useful way.

Other mealtime behaviors *are* connected to food itself and, surprisingly, appear to be nearly universal. For instance:

No Touching Allowed. Most children pass through a stage in which they will not eat foods that have touched other foods. A child might like mashed potatoes and meat loaf but will not eat either if they've come into contact with one another. Trying to get a child in this stage to eat a casserole may create a conflict. *Recommendation:* Serve one food at a time or provide a compartmentalized plate that keeps foods from spilling into each other.

Food Jags. Another common behavior is the "food jag," in which a child will eat one and only one food, meal after meal. Parents of children who refuse any variety in their diets worry that their child is being malnourished. Though the jags seem to last forever, they rarely last long enough to cause real harm. *Recommendation:* If your child will eat

THE NUTRITIONAL NEEDS OF CHILDREN

nothing but peanut butter sandwiches, for example, give him one for every lunchtime meal. At breakfast, offer him a quarter of a sandwich with some other selections, such as milk and a piece of fruit. You can try the same approach for dinner, offering part of a sandwich along with the rest of the meal.

After a few days, it is likely that he'll experiment with other foods. This is *not* the time to try to remove peanut butter sandwiches from the table. Instead, offer the sandwich for as long as he wants it. One day, to your surprise, he'll declare that he *hates* peanut butter—and *loves* tuna fish.

Plain Is Perfect. Many children pass through a stage in which they want their food "naked"—no sauce, no spices, nothing to disguise the essential food. Since their taste buds are much more acute than those of adults, added flavorings can be overpowering. *Recommendation:* When preparing a meal that you prefer with a sauce, place the sauce in a separate serving bowl from which kids can try a bit if they'd like.

Try It. Color, texture, appearance, smell, and even how a food feels inside his mouth are all considerations a child makes before trying new foods. Untried red foods, which are most often sweet, for instance, may be more readily accepted than untried green foods, which the child has associated with bitter tastes. Unusual textures and hard-to-chew foods, such as meat, may not appeal to toddlers. For reasons that are not clear, American children are more likely to try carrots, broccoli, pepper, and other vegetables raw rather than cooked. Both the mushy texture and the smell of cooked vegetables are a "turnoff." (Interestingly, in other cultures such as India, where soft vegetables are a mainstay, children show no aversion to either the texture or the smell of cooked vegetables.) *Recommendation:* Don't pressure children into trying new foods. Rather, offer a variety, relax, and eventually you'll be more likely to hear complaints about not enough variety!

Source: From *The Yummy or Yucky Taste Test,* by Jo-Ann Heslin, M.A., R.D. and Annette Natow, Ph.D., R.D. Reprinted from *Sesame Street Magazine Parents' Guide,* April 1988.

● ●

CHAPTER SEVEN

......

The Nutritional Needs of Preschoolers

Between the ages of three and five, a child masters almost all of the basic eating skills. Her full set of first teeth allows her to master the art of chewing, and increasing dexterity enables her to learn to use a spoon and fork with relative ease. Using a knife to cut food may still require further practice, but most four- or five-year-olds can become adept at using a dull-bladed knife to spread food, such as peanut butter, onto a slice of bread. And while they have mastered the art of drinking from a cup or glass, it will still be a while before they can be counted on not to spill their milk with incredible frequency. By this age, too, most children are ready to learn some basic table manners.

Preschoolers are still in a period of slow growth. They increase their weight by only about 12 percent between the ages of three and five, although you will see quite a change in their appearance as their bodies stretch and slim down.

Most preschoolers eat only very small amounts of food—distressingly small by some adult standards. This habit concerns and puzzles many parents, since their children seem healthy and full of energy. When children seem healthy, they usually are, which should be a relief to parents. In any case, children at this age like to eat when they are hungry, and they usually stop eating when they are full. This is to be encouraged, for being attuned to the body's needs at a young age can mark the beginning of a lifetime of good eating habits.

What to Feed Them

By age four, preschoolers are usually able to eat everything that the rest of the family can handle. Their tastes usually broaden significantly as their curiosity spurs them to try new things, but the favorites during this period are still likely to be the old standbys, especially hamburgers and spaghetti. They'll still need a few substantial snacks a day, and you can make sure these snacks are nutritious rather than just sweet and filling, by keeping foods such as crackers or bread with cheese or peanut butter, hard-boiled eggs, raw vegetables, fresh fruit and fruit juice, milk, yogurt, and pudding on hand.

The characteristic independence of preschoolers is complemented by an eagerness to be a part of the adult world. Finally able to sit at the dinner table, preschoolers are generally able (and often determined!) to take part in the family meal. They are also often willing and eager to help around the house, in the yard—and in the kitchen. Preschoolers take great pleasure in serving themselves at the table, although not consistently. At some meals, they will insist they can do everything themselves, and at other times they will seem to regress, requiring a lot of attention and help to get through a meal, perhaps needing to be excused early.

Another common characteristic among preschoolers is a certain susceptibility to what they see and hear around them. The good news is that they begin to copy the good behavior they see; the bad news is that they start listening to advertising—both from TV and from their friends. All of a sudden, you may find that your child, who once snacked on nothing but fresh fruit, can't live a moment longer without a presweetened crunchy munchy. Thus, long before your child knows the capital of the state you're living in, she knows exactly what kind of cereal or cookie she wants.

All is not lost. The preschool years are the ideal time to begin teaching the principles of sound nutrition in a conscious and conscientious way. Children of this age are receptive and willing to share your point of view—particularly if you make the learning process fun. Having your child help wash, dice, and slice casserole ingredients, for instance, can have many rewards: She learns to understand that wholes are made up of parts, she practices manual dexterity, and, best of all, she gets to spend time with you. You can sometimes reason with preschoolers, too, explaining that the foods you want them to eat will make them healthy and strong while some of the foods advertised on TV may not be as good for them. And you can, without fear of throwing years of good nutrition down the drain, allow some ''junk food'' into the house. The benefit of this approach is that you don't encourage her to overvalue a food by making it off-limits.

Preschoolers' eating preferences and habits also reflect their sense of independence. Like toddlers, they are subject to food quirks (see pages 95–97). And like children at any age, their tastes are forever changing. Thus, a problem that exists today is unlikely to persist for long. Ultimately, the most important step you can take in determine your preschooler's eating patterns is to set a good example yourself.

The following graphs will give you some idea of the heights and weights of the average child from age two through age eighteen:

GIRLS FROM 2 TO 18 YEARS
WEIGHT FOR AGE

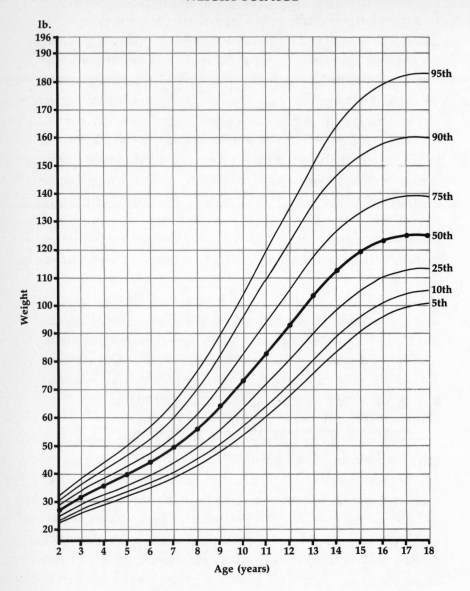

Source: Department of Health, Education and Welfare, Public Health Service, Health Resources Administration, National Center for Health Statistics, and Center for Disease Control.

BOYS FROM 2 TO 18 YEARS
WEIGHT FOR AGE

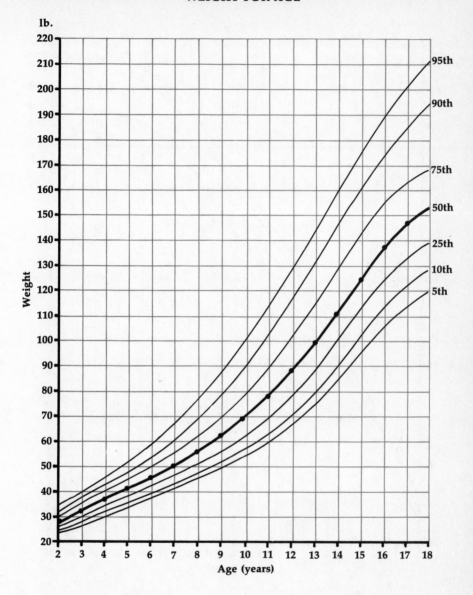

Source: Department of Health, Education and Welfare, Public Health Service, Health Resources Administration, National Center for Health Statistics, and Center for Disease Control.

GIRLS FROM 2 TO 18 YEARS
STATURE FOR AGE

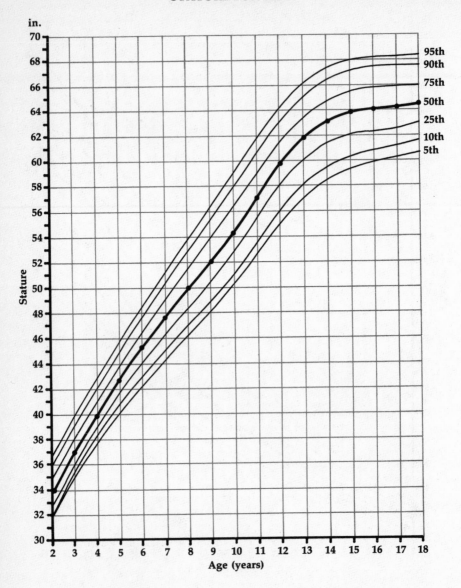

Source: Department of Health, Education and Welfare, Public Health Service, Health Resources Administration, National Center for Health Statistics, and Center for Disease Control.

BOYS FROM 2 TO 18 YEARS
STATURE FOR AGE

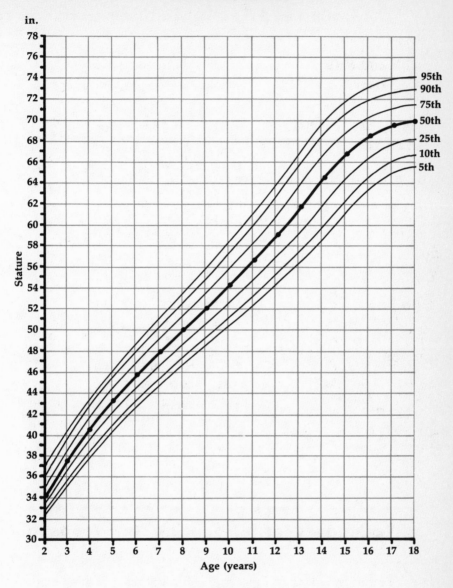

Source: Department of Health, Education and Welfare, Public Health Service, Health Resources Administration, National Center for Health Statistics, and Center for Disease Control.

• •

The Daily Food Needs of Preschoolers

Milk and Milk Products:
Four to six $\frac{1}{2}$-cup servings of whole milk, yogurt, or buttermilk

Meat, Fish, Poultry, and Other High-Protein Foods:
Three 1-ounce servings of meat, fish, poultry, eggs, cheese, tofu, peanut butter, or legumes

Fruits and Vegetables:
Four or more $\frac{1}{4}$-cup servings, at least one of which should be rich in vitamin C and another rich in vitamin A

Grains:
Four servings
- One serving of bread is $\frac{1}{2}$ slice.
- One serving of cereal or pasta is $\frac{1}{2}$ cup, cooked.
- One serving of breakfast cereal is $\frac{1}{2}$ cup.

Source: *No-Nonsense Nutrition for Kids*, by Annette B. Natow and Jo-Ann Heslin, copyright ©, 1984. Published by McGraw-Hill, Inc. Used with permission of authors.

• •

Techniques for Introducing New Foods

- Encourage kids to share in food preparation, including menu planning and cooking.

- Offer untried foods alongside familiar foods. For example, a child who likes yogurt may be willing to try a new vegetable that's served with a yogurt dip.

- Sandwich bread is a good "holder" for new foods. Try cutting bread into fun shapes.

- "Draw" a smiling face on top of a casserole, using strips of cheese cut-outs or some other familiar food.

- Encourage a child to try a bite; never insist that she eat more than a taste. (If she spits it out, refrain from getting angry. Instead, say, "I guess this is something you'll like when you're a little older.")

- Let your child know when you're trying something new to eat. Share the stories of your own childhood food dislikes, too.

- Relax.

• •
How Other Caregivers Can Help Your Children

One of the first places you are likely to come across eating patterns contrary to your own is at a day-care center or a baby-sitter's home. Many caregivers are aware of good nutrition and the eating habits of young children, but not all of them may be as knowledgeable or as scrupulous about nutrition as you would like. The best way to determine a center's nutritional philosophy is to ask questions and observe. If fresh fruit is served at snacktime and sandwiches are made from whole-grain breads, you can probably rest assured that they won't be feeding children high-fat, overly processed, or overly sugary foods. Ask for a listing of snacks and meals they normally provide.

If what you hear and see doesn't make you happy, you can (tactfully) ask for their reasons for serving food less nutritious than you would like. If it's a matter of lack of knowledge, you can offer to help them restructure their program. If there is no way to change the system, you can ask if your children may bring their own food. (If the answer is yes, make sure such meals take little preparation; asking the caretaker to assume the task of preparing or cooking something complicated isn't reasonable, particularly if he or she is responsible for several children.) Remember, though, that while eating food from home can work well with infants and toddlers, the plan may backfire with preschoolers, who may feel singled out and self-conscious.

Consider how many meals your child will actually eat away from home. She will probably be eating at least one or two, perhaps even three meals (midmorning snack, lunch, afternoon snack) if she's there all day. Partly on that basis, you can make the decision about how important the issue is to you. If it's just a snack or lunch, you might compromise, figuring that the good breakfast, dinner, and other snacks you provide and the habits you teach at home will make up for a few less-than-perfect meals.

If a sitter comes to your home, you can expect the person to follow your wishes entirely, with some qualifications. You can't reasonably expect a sitter to make elaborate preparations unless she particularly likes to, but you can expect that your basic guidelines will be followed. Make sure you outline your wishes, since older children, from preschool on, are not always the most accurate sources of information about the foods that you allow.

When it comes to grandparents, other relatives, and friends, you may have to be more diplomatic when you come across different food attitudes. Ask them to respect your wishes when your child is with them. Explain to them why you are teaching your children to eat nutritionally sound foods. Then relax. Don't let this issue become a battleground in itself or an excuse to battle over other, unspoken, issues, and don't be afraid to compromise. Their theories on feeding children, while perhaps different from yours, are based on a lifetime of firmly held ideas. If they want to feed your child candy occasionally, it won't do her any permanent harm, and can, in fact, have emotional benefits to grandparents who enjoy indulging and to children who enjoy being indulged. The opposite scenario is also possible: For example, you may allow frozen juice pops for breakfast as a substitute for juice, which can cause alarm in your child's grandparent. The bottom line is that it's more important for your child to develop a good relationship with her relatives than it is to devote much time and energy into arguments about food.

● ●

CHAPTER EIGHT

· · · · · ·

The Nutritional Needs of Grade-Schoolers

The first day of school is a momentous occasion for all parents; it's hard not to get a little teary-eyed as you see your small son or daughter going off into the Real World without you. Among other things, who knows *what* they'll eat out there?

The grade-school years are a period of relatively modest growth among children. Proportionally, their nutritional needs for protein and certain fundamental vitamins and minerals, such as vitamins C and D, calcium, phosphorus, iron, and zinc, are basically the same as those of a four-year-old. Of course, a ten-year-old needs a larger quantity of food than a preschooler for his larger body. The amount of food necessary for a child of this age will vary with the individual child, but the balance will be the same for every grade-schooler. The emphasis should be on complex carbohydrates—fruits, vegetables, whole grains, and breads—followed by fats, and then proteins. (The balance translates into a diet in which about 55 percent of the calories come from carbohydrates, 30 percent from fats, and 15 percent from proteins.)

The basic eating skills of children become very well developed during this period. First-graders may have trouble

THE NUTRITIONAL NEEDS OF CHILDREN

cutting their own food, perhaps needing help for another year or two, but by age eight or nine, children will be deftly using most eating utensils.

School-age children in particular need a good breakfast to keep them alert for that long haul until lunch. Children who have eaten a good breakfast have been shown to be less fidgety and better able to concentrate and tackle problems then those who have not. It's particularly important for first-graders to eat a complete breakfast, since the mid-morning snack to which most of them are accustomed suddenly ceases to arrive. A balanced breakfast containing a high-protein food along with fruit and bread is ideal. Cereal with milk, juice or fruit, and toast make up the standard meal, but you don't have to be bound by convention. There is nothing wrong with a cheese or meat loaf sandwich or any other nutritious food or combination that kids will actually eat. Not every child has an appetite for a large breakfast, but even a glass of milk or a carton of yogurt can give him a good start. If it takes him a while to work up an appetite, send him off with a sandwich that can be eaten on the way to school or just before the first bell rings.

The figures on the graph on pages 102–105 will give you some idea of what to expect in the way of growth in your grade-school-age child.

Food Freedom

One of the main differences in eating habits to emerge during the grade-school years is a desire for what might be called "food freedom," which is another way of saying that what Mom and Dad don't know about what you eat won't hurt them. During first grade, a child will probably take a lunch prepared from home and eat it dutifully and without question. However, as he becomes more comfortable with his peers and his newfound freedom, he may begin to exert some initiative. Be prepared for the discovery that the wholesome lunch you provide may not be eaten quite as you planned. Children often swap parts of their lunches at school or eat only the parts that appeal to them and pitch the rest.

Expressions of food freedom may cause your child to dictate very precisely what will go into his lunch box. Unless his requests are ludicrous, it is probably a good idea to give him what he wants. Getting him to help make the lunch may help ensure that he eats it, too. Be prepared for dramatic changes in the menu, however. His favorite lunch for years may have been a peanut butter and jelly sandwich on whole wheat bread, carrot sticks, and an apple. Then one day he'll change his order to a bologna sandwich on white with mustard—something he would never have dreamed of touching before. It may be that his tastes have changed. It may also be that peer pressure is taking over. It's a good idea to respect his wishes while seeking some sort of compromise.

Grade-school children respond not just to their friends but also to the lure of vending machines and candy shops. As they learn to handle money, they also learn to spend it, often on what writer Vicki Lansky calls Constantly Advertised Nutritionally Deficient Yummies (C.A.N.D.Y.). Children with reasonably sound eating habits won't be harmed by the occasional chocolate bar, and forbidding children to buy such treats can cause more problems than it solves by making these foods seem more glamorous and desirable than they are. Reasoning with grade-schoolers sometimes works, but a key strategy is to provide nutritious food at home and set a good example by not indulging in high-fat, high-sugar treats yourself. Establish sensible, realistic rules: one piece of candy a day, or one a week, or only at home, where a child can brush his teeth right after he eats sweets, for example. These policies are not easy to enforce—but that shouldn't keep you from trying.

Your child may also become more vocal now about wanting you to stock up on some packaged foods that he sees advertised on television and elsewhere. How you handle insistent requests for such treats is an individual matter. One mother had a particularly ingenious solution: When her son had driven her to virtual distraction with his requests for a sugary cereal, she finally gave in and bought a box, on one condition: He was not allowed to have the cereal for breakfast; he could, however, eat it for dessert. By reaching this compromise, she was able to reinforce her message that breakfast be more nutritious while allowing her son to make a reasonable choice. No one ''lost face.'' Parental authority and a child's need for autonomy were both honored.

Just as preschoolers need small extra meals, grade-schoolers need to supplement their three squares with snacks. The time-honored, after-school snack need not turn into an all-afternoon affair, however, and some attempt to make it nutritious should be made. Some satisfying healthful snacks include a piece of fruit, a serving of flavored yogurt, a piece of bread with peanut butter, a slice of cheese and a couple of crackers, or a serving of leftovers from dinner the night before.

If your family routine includes eating dinner together at the table at a set time, you will probably want to limit the size of the after-school snack. To keep a snack from growing into a marathon eating session, encourage kids to treat it like a small meal, eaten from a plate on the table. An open box of crackers or a large container of dried fruit placed on the coffee table in front of the TV is an invitation for the child to keep eating without giving any thought to the process. Children of this age are quite capable of getting their own snacks, and indeed they should be encouraged to take some responsibility. This doesn't mean they should have carte blanche when it comes to snacking. A cookie here, a little sandwich there, a piece of fruit, and a glass of milk throughout the afternoon add up to a lot of food. Children can take the responsibility of serving themselves, but they should not be encouraged to get so full that they won't eat and enjoy their dinner. This is an age at which you can begin to teach children to be responsible for what they eat. The habits they form now will be with them for a lifetime.

The grade-school years are a good time to begin involving children in actual cooking—not just acting as your kitchen helper but actually mastering some cooking techniques. Both boys and girls in the middle-school years often enjoy developing their own specialties, too.

Don't expect grade-schoolers to develop gourmet tastes. They may still separate each food on a plate, and they will probably pick out the onions or other "icky" things in a dish. These peculiarities will pass eventually. Before you know it, your child will come home from school and ask if you know how to make broiled mushroom caps.

● ●

The Daily Food Needs of Grade-Schoolers

Milk and Milk Products:	Two or three 1-cup servings
Meat, Fish, Poultry, and Other High-Protein Foods:	Two 2-ounce servings

Fruits and Vegetables: Four or more ¹/₂-cup servings, including one serving rich in vita-
min C and one rich in vitamin A
• One medium-size piece of fruit
is one serving.

Grains: Four servings
• One serving of bread is 1 slice.
• One serving of cereal, rice, or
pasta is ¹/₂ cup, cooked.

Source: No-Nonsense Nutrition for Kids, by Annette B. Natow and Jo-Ann Heslin, copyright ©,
1984. Published by McGraw-Hill, Inc. Used with permission of authors.

• •

School Lunch Programs

Once children reach grade school, it becomes much more of a
challenge to monitor their schooltime diets. Not only do you
need to know what the school is serving in its lunch program;
you have to think about what the other kids are eating as well.
There's nothing you can do about the lunches that other children bring to school, of course, but you can and should inves-
tigate what is being offered by your child's school cafeteria.

If your child's school is a member of the National School
Lunch Program, a federally funded program, the lunch provided
each day is designed to meet one third of a child's daily nutritional needs. It consists of five foods from the four food groups
and must contain 2 ounces of meat or meat substitute, ³/₄ cup
of fruit, ³/₄ cup of vegetables, one serving of a whole-grain or
enriched-grain product (bread, pasta, rice, or noodles), and one
serving of milk. In some schools, a child is allowed to forgo
either the milk or the fruit or vegetables. This rule has been

established to avoid some of the waste that occurs when children throw away the foods they won't touch.

Increasingly, however, the services that provide cafeteria meals are under pressure to be profitable. Becoming profitable means that the food provided has to be popular enough for children to want it and inexpensive enough for the service to be able to provide it at a reasonable price. What can happen is that the school system turns to fast-food-style lunches that are high in fat and sodium but low in other essential nutrients. Some schools also have vending machines for soda, candy, and sweet snacks.

What can a parent do? Begin by voicing your concern. If possible, enlist the aid of other parents. If enough parents present their views, school officials are likely to respond positively.

As a child goes out into the world, perhaps the best piece of advice a parent can embrace is to change what you can, accept what you can't change, and provide good food and a good example at home.

• •

CHAPTER NINE

......

The Nutritional Needs of Preteens

If you want to know what variety is, take a look at a group of thirty twelve-year-olds. They come in all shapes and sizes. For many children, particularly girls, the years eleven and twelve signal the beginning of their last major growth spurt. This period of growth usually continues into the teen years, but most girls reach the peak of growth at around age twelve. Boys begin their intensive growth a little later; about half of them are into it by age twelve, and most reach their growth peaks at about age fifteen.

The preteen years are a time when the body begins to go through its most dramatic changes to date and when a child's perception of herself in relation to her body becomes of paramount importance. The beginning of the growth spurt signals the start of all kinds of changes, including increased nutritional needs. In fact, children need more food during these years of intense growth than at any other time in their lives.

Preteens who participate in sports have especially increased energy needs and thus have an increased need for foods rich in complex carbohydrates, such as breads, pasta, rice, and potatoes, which provide easily used energy and needed vitamins.

The Importance of Iron and Calcium to Preteens

Since girls do most of their growing during early adolescence, they need to be particularly careful to eat enough nutritious foods during this period. Their iron needs, for example, increase as a result of the onset of menstruation (usually between ages twelve and thirteen), so they need to eat plenty of iron-rich foods. Girls and boys from age eleven to eighteen need about 18 milligrams of iron daily, or the amount found in a balanced diet of about 3,000 calories a day. Growing boys have no trouble eating that much and more (much more), but girls, who may be starting to worry about their weight and possibly putting themselves on weight-reducing diets, may have a problem getting the iron they need and may need iron supplements. To get enough iron from their diets alone, they should eat iron-rich foods, including liver (not usually a preteen's first menu choice), turkey, beef, pork, beans, and prunes. If they shun these foods, they can also get by eating iron-enriched flours and cereals. (For a list of other iron-rich foods, see pages 31–32.)

To accommodate their growing bones, both boys and girls need to increase their intake of calcium during the critical preteen years. Girls in particular need to be sure to eat foods rich in calcium. Unfortunately, however, this is a time when some teens are beginning to resist drinking milk, thinking of it as babyish or possibly fattening. By this age, it is perfectly appropriate for them to drink low-fat or skim milk. If you can't persuade eleven- and twelve-year-olds to drink milk regularly, encourage them to try other calcium-rich foods. (For a list of foods high in calcium, see pages 29–30.)

The changes that take place in preteens are not just physical; the preteen years are marked by emotional upheaveals, too. In addition to disrupting eating patterns, these emotional highs and lows can have an effect on nutrition. Emotional stress can interfere with the body's ability to use nutrients, especially calcium, protein, and vitamins A and C.

Peer Pressure

Even more than grade-schoolers, preteens are influenced by their friends at school. It's vitally important to most preteens to seem grown-up, and one of the easiest ways they can manage this is to change their eating habits, not always for the better. Gone are the milk, juice, and water they used to drink with meals; now they may opt for sugary soft drinks. Preadolescent girls who become extremely body-conscious sometimes drink diet soft drinks to the exclusion of all other beverages. Sodas in general have little nutritional benefit, except for the energy of the sugar they contain, and when they're made with artificial sweeteners, they are deprived of even that. In addition, there is some evidence that Aspartame, a commonly used artificial sweetener, may trigger migraine headaches in those prone to this condition. The phosphorus found in many carbonated soft drinks can also inhibit the absorption of calcium from foods.

Encourage your preteen to drink soda sparingly and never with meals. Keep offering low-fat milk, juice, and water. If all else fails, try suggesting that if they really want to be sophisticated, they'll drink mineral water or seltzer.

Getting Your Kids Involved

Nutritionally speaking, the best thing parents can do during the preteen years is to provide healthful meals at home and encourage their kids to stay home as often as possible to eat them.

If your child has eaten sensibly all her life, she may get through this time without much of a problem. However, no matter how well some kids have been taught, they may use their newfound freedom to throw reason and good sense to the wind. If that happens, the best thing a parent can do is to avoid nagging. (This is also the hardest thing to do.) Just because a child doesn't do the right thing doesn't mean she's forgotten what the right thing is. Be patient. She's likely to return eventually to the eating habits you helped her develop earlier.

To speed up that return, try involving a child in healthful nutrition by appealing to his or her developing body sense. If you can get across the idea that good nutrition offers a way to create a good-looking or strong body, you will have won an important battle. Don't forget: Fitness is downright fashionable among teens. You might want to encourage other significant people in your child's life to lend a hand, since preteens look to teenagers and other older people as role models. Coaches and older siblings are often invested with more authority than parents, and if they take a position that eating a balanced diet will improve performance or appearance, preteens are more likely to listen.

Another good method for involving preteens in healthful eating is to make food preparation part of the regular household routine. Take your child grocery shopping; encourage her to help with certain food-preparation tasks; give her responsibility for planning and preparing at least one evening meal every week. As long as it's a well-balanced meal, let her make whatever she likes. A cheeseburger, broccoli, and lime Jell-O may not be your idea of a perfect meal, but if it's hers, so be it.

Many preteens, both boys and girls, take cooking classes in school, and bringing their skills home is a good way of reinforcing good eating habits.

Eating Away from Home

Preteens spend a lot of time away from home, and many parents worry that they spend most of it eating french fries and drinking cola. They eat more snacks and meals at friends' houses or out after games or club meetings. Fast food is a particular favorite, along with the sweets of earlier childhood. There is little parents can do to control what foods a child eats away from home, nor should they try too hard. All you can do is make the child understand how you feel about empty-calorie food and take even more care to see that the meals and snacks that are eaten at home are well-rounded and nutritious.

• •

The Daily Food Needs of Preteens

Milk and Milk Products: Two to three 1-cup servings

Meat, Fish, Poultry, and Other High-Protein Foods: Three 2-ounce servings

Fruits and Vegetables: Four or more servings, including at least one serving of fruit or vegetables rich in vitamin C and one serving rich in vitamin A
- One serving of a vegetable is ½ cup.
- One serving of fruit is ½ cup cooked or canned fruit or 1 medium piece of fresh fruit.

Grains: Four or more servings
- One serving of bread is 1 slice.
- One serving of cooked and dry cereal, rice, or pasta is ½ cup.

Source: *No-Nonsense Nutrition for Kids,* by Annette B. Natow and Jo-Ann Heslin, copyright © 1984. Published by McGraw-Hill, Inc. Used with permission of authors.

• •

CHAPTER TEN

• • • • • •

The Nutritional Needs of Teens

If you wake up one morning and discover that there's not a scrap of food in the house even though you went shopping only yesterday, chances are good that you're the parent of a teenager. Many people remember the teen years as a time of endless appetite. Boys, in particular, suddenly seem capable of emptying a refrigerator in one sitting, eating the family dinner fixings and all the breakfast food in the process. Most boys and many girls at this age are able to eat huge quantities of food without gaining excess weight. This is particularly true of teens who are active in sports.

Like the first year of life, the teen years are a period of intense growth. Children who were sort of plump tend to stretch up and grow with alarming speed. Boys often grow several inches a year, requiring new clothes every few months. Girls take on curves and a new softness.

Boys and girls grow at noticeably different rates during adolescence. Girls begin their growth spurt at about ten or eleven, peak at around twelve, and usually finish by fifteen. Boys begin theirs at twelve or thirteen, peak at about fifteen, and stop at around nineteen. These growth spurts usually account for almost 50 percent of their adult weight. It's hardly surprising, given the rapid growth and changes that occur and the demands made by increased activity, that the food needs of teens increase along with their appetites.

It's not just the timing of the growth spurts that differs between boys and girls. Boys add mostly muscle and bone tissue during this intense growth spurt, ending up with about 8 percent body fat. Girls add proportionately more fat, reaching about 20 percent. This fat level has more to do with hormones than with food and physical activity. No matter what the reason, though, girls need fewer calories than boys do, even if their weights are the same. A typical adolescent boy will need about 3,000 calories a day, while a girl of the same age will require about 2,200. Many of their nutritional needs remain the same, however; both continue to require similar amounts of calcium, zinc, phosphorus, iodine, vitamins C and D, certain B vitamins, and folacin.

Like all children, adolescents grow at varying rates; the graphs on pages 102–105 give a general idea of the average heights and weights of teenagers.

Special Nutritional Needs of Teens

The increased need for food by teens is also accompanied, many parents find, by the end of any control they have over their children's diets. Teenagers are even more independent than their younger siblings, spending increased amounts of time with friends, arranging their own meals, and often eating out.

On those increasingly rare occasions when you do have something to say about what your teenager eats, continue to stress a well-rounded diet, rich in a variety of nutrients from meat and other protein-rich foods, dairy products, fruits and vegetables, and breads and grains. Pay special attention to your teenager's intake of calcium, vitamin D, and iron.

Teenagers need lots of calcium to build strong bones. During preadolescence, most children drink milk and eat dairy products with little complaint. During the preteen and teen years, however, they tend to favor carbonated soft drinks, sometimes exclusively. The problem is not just that they contain lots of sugar or artificial sweeteners, which they certainly do; it's also that they contain large amounts of phosphorus, which reduces the body's ability to process calcium. The Recommended Daily Allowance (RDA) of calcium is roughly 1,200 milligrams per day, the amount in four 8-ounce glasses of milk (whole, low-fat, or skim) or containers of yogurt. The vitamin D found in fortified milk also helps the body absorb calcium. (See pages 29–30 for a list of calcium-rich foods.) Ice cream and fast-food shakes that are made with milk also contain calcium, but again, they have less calcium than plain milk, and they're very high in fat and sugar.

Teenage boys and girls need plenty of iron, too, since they are still building body tissue and blood. Once girls begin to menstruate, they also need to replace the iron lost during menstruation. (See pages 31–32 for a list of iron-rich foods.)

Iron deficiency sometimes becomes a problem during adolescence, particularly for girls, who tend to go on fad diets to control their weight, but also for boys, whose appetites may not keep pace with their rapid growth. Boys and girls should both consume about 18 milligrams of iron a day to avoid iron-deficiency anemia, the symptoms of which are a lack of energy and a quickness to fatigue, pale skin, and frequent infections. If eating enough iron-rich foods just isn't possible, an iron supplement may be called for, but only after consulting a health professional.

How Much?

Just how much does the average adolescent need to eat? The answer is fairly simple: A teenage boy needs the equivalent of four square meals a day—four or more servings of milk products, fruit and vegetables, and bread and cereal; and three or more servings of meat or other protein-rich foods—and a teenage girl needs a solid three. All of this food may be consumed as actual meals or as meals supplemented with snacks. Most teens prefer the snack approach. Unlike younger children, most fast-growing teenagers who snack frequently are also able to eat full meals when the time comes. The goal, of course, is to get them to snack on foods high in nutrients, not just high in energy (such as sugary or fatty treats). Some good snack foods are fresh fruit, crackers, popcorn, sandwiches, cheese, and yogurt.

During growth spurts, some teens will need even more than the above-mentioned quantities of food.

Eating Habits

Where did you go wrong? You've tried your best to teach your child how to eat right; you've given him only the best foods, prepared in the most healthful way; you've taught him the difference between nutritious and empty-calorie snacks. How come he's up in his room right now eating his own weight in taco-flavored corn chips and washing them down with root beer? The first thing to remember is not to take it personally.

The eating habits of teenagers are almost completely of their own choosing, and frequently, they are in direct conflict with the teachings of their childhoods. This doesn't mean, however, that you've done something wrong if suddenly all your son wants is pizza, morning, noon, and night. In the first place, pizza isn't the worst choice of foods. Second, what he eats is his choice now, not yours. You can still set a good example and prepare balanced meals, and it's reasonable to expect that even a teenager will eat dinner with his family. Other than that, you can just keep your fingers crossed and hope that there is enough variety amid the quantity of the food he is eating to keep him healthy.

Having a role in the preparation of family meals can be of great value to the teenager. As discussed in previous chapters, if a child is given responsibility in shopping for or fixing meals, nutritional teachings will be more deeply ingrained. By the teen years, kids are quite capable of taking on the responsibility of preparing meals. Indeed, in a national survey conducted by Teenage Research Unlimited during June and July of 1987, 80 percent of the 2,200 teenagers polled said they had made a meal for themselves in the previous week. Some teens cook because there is no one at home to do it for them; others cook simply because they like to.

● ●

The Nutritional Value of Teen-Pleasing Foods

Teens like to eat out, and for most of them this translates into fast food. Take comfort: Fast foods aren't devoid of nutritional value; indeed, they contain many of the nutrients a child needs. The combination of a hamburger, fries, and a shake, for instance, derives 17 percent of its calories from protein, 39 percent from fat, and 44 percent from carbohydrates. This is not too bad a balance, all things considered, though it's rather high on the fat side. (Remember, the ideal proportions are 15 percent protein, 30 percent fat, and 55 percent carbohydrates.) Fruits and vegetables aren't in great abundance in such a meal, but then again, you don't have to have fruits and vegetables at every meal. Another teen favorite, pizza, is actually a pretty healthful food. A typical slice contains about 15 percent protein, 27 percent fat, and 58 percent carbohydrates. You wouldn't want your child to eat every meal at a fast-food establishment, but neither the hamburger stand nor the pizza joint is a total loss in terms of nutrition.

Acne

For years, diet has been blamed for outbreaks of acne in adolescents, and certain foods have been branded as chronic offenders. Most commonly cited were chocolate and fried foods. However, recent research shows that diet has little or nothing to do with causing acne. Acne is caused, quite simply, by hormonal activity that alters the skin's normal processes. It can be exacerbated by grease left on the face after eating greasy foods. Thus, a child who eats French fries should wash his face and hands thoroughly to avoid leaving a greasy residue on his face.

The only known dietary factor related to acne is that deficiencies in vitamin A and zinc can make an outbreak of acne worse. A reasonably well balanced diet, however, will give a teen all the vitamin A and zinc he needs.

• •
The Daily Food Needs of Teenagers

Boys in periods of active growth may need more food than the portions noted below. Girls whose growth has begun to slow may need a little less.

Milk and Milk Products:

Four 1-cup servings

Meat, Fish, Poultry, and Other High-Protein Foods:

Three or more 2-ounce servings

Fruits and Vegetables:

Four or more ½-cup servings, including one rich in vitamin C and one rich in vitamin A
- 1 medium-size fruit is one serving.

Grains:

Four or more servings
- One serving of bread is 1 slice.
- One serving of cereal, rice, or pasta is ½ cup.

Source: No-Nonsense Nutrition for Kids, by Annette B. Natow and Jo-Ann Heslin, copyright © 1984. Published by McGraw-Hill, Inc. Used with permission of authors.
• •

Special Section:
Eating Disorders

• • • • • •

In a study of girls' dieting habits, University of Michigan researchers found that 36 percent of girls between the ages of nine and twenty were on a diet. Among the ten- and eleven-year-olds, 23 percent of the girls were trying to reduce. Almost all adolescent girls feel that they are not as slim as the models in print ads, movies, and television who define today's concept of beauty.

Most adolescent girls, in fact, are not fat, but it's just about impossible to get some of them to believe it. Parents' best strategy is not to overreact to a child's actions and not to set a bad example by being obsessed with weight. Try to keep teenagers interested in as many foods as possible and instill in them some sense of balance.

For those teenagers who are more than 15 percent overweight or underweight, this is the time to reinforce good nutritional habits. And for those teenagers who show signs of taking dieting too seriously, be aware of the possibility that they may have a serious eating disorder. The two most serious, and increasingly common, disorders are *anorexia nervosa* and *bulimia*.

Anorexia Nervosa

Victims of anorexia feel that they can never be thin enough, and they deprive themselves of food, even when it is easily available. If left untreated, anorexics can literally starve themselves to death. Anorexia works against the normal bodily functions, because the victim's normal signals to eat, such as appetite and hunger, no longer function properly. Eventually children, even extraordinarily hungry children, *cannot* eat.

No one knows why some children and young adults are affected with the disorder and others aren't. The various clues do not add up to a coherent picture of the problem, and it's quite possible that there will never be a clear-cut answer. What we do know is that it's a disorder having to do with growing up and the uncertainties it causes. It is far more common in girls than in boys. Occasionally, adult women and men develop anorexia nervosa, but it's much more common in adolescents and usually begins a year or two after a child has reached puberty. It seems to be a way of retreating from the frightening uncertainties of growing up, a means of gaining control over their lives, and a way to keep the body from maturing. (It works, too. Menstruation stops after the body's fat stores are depleted. The reduced fat stores also mean that girls lose their rounded breasts, hips, and calves.)

Anorexia nervosa victims are not consciously trying to hurt themselves or their families. They are often compliant in all other areas of family life.

Signs to Look for

Lots of teenagers go on diets for one reason or another. Practically all of them come off them shortly, regardless of whether they have reached their desired weight. Sometimes those who develop anorexia start by dieting very successfully, losing all the weight they had planned. However, they don't stop there; they go on, never satisfied with their degree of thinness.

Anorexia is not something a child comes down with today and for which she can be treated tomorrow. It is a progressive disorder, one that even experts do not always recognize at first. There are, however, certain signs to look for:

1. If a child loses an extreme amount of weight, you should keep a close eye on her. The weight loss doesn't mean she definitely is anorexic, but it does mean her condition bears watching. If your child is within 10 percent of the average weight for a girl of her age and height, she's probably okay, provided she doesn't continue to lose weight. If a girl's current weight is 15 percent below normal, you have cause for concern. When her weight reaches 20 percent below normal, her health will be affected.

2. If your daughter's menstruation has stopped in addition to her undergoing severe weight loss, you should be concerned. She may not be menstruating for a number of other reasons, but you should be aware of the problem. In any case, she needs medical help.

3. Consider your child's attitudes toward food. A teen with anorexia may exhibit habits that suggest she is avoiding food, such as deleting all high-carbohydrate foods and fats from her diet, serving herself tiny portions, and

avoiding all snacks. These appear to be the habits of a conscientious dieter, but when a child is already too thin, they can be considered symptoms of anorexia.

4. Those with anorexia are usually fascinated with food. Often they will gladly cook but won't eat the food they prepare. They are usually obsessed with the way other people look, finding the least amount of fat on someone very distasteful. They often hang around supermarkets and food shops and spend lots of the time in the kitchen during meal preparation.

5. Many anorexics are interested in fitness to the extreme. Some are aspiring athletes. Even when they lose muscle mass as a result of starvation, they put great physical demands on their bodies with vigorous exercise.

6. Occasionally, the body overwhelms anorexics, and they binge on food. Having allowed themselves to taste something, they then can't stop themselves and eat a very large, sometimes huge quantity, such as an entire bunch of broccoli or two or three pints of ice cream. Sometimes these food "binges" are minor, confined to picking at leftovers or licking mixing spoons. Always, though, after one of these "slips" the anorexic becomes more rigid with herself, eating even less.

If you recognize all or some of these signs in your daughter or son, get help immediately. Don't just hope it will all get better; confront the issue head-on. Talk it over with your child. If she promises to do better, give her a little time to do so. There is a chance she may be able to get over it with encouragement. But don't wait too long. If she doesn't gain weight within a week or two (watch out for sneaky behavior such as drinking lots of water before weighing in, weighting her pockets, or taking laxatives after weighing in), seek professional help. Your child's physical condition will need attention, so the first step is to treat the physical symptoms with proper medical care. The next step is to treat the psychological causes of the behavior.

Medical doctors and mental-health professionals specializing in adolescents are increasingly aware of the problem, and numerous programs have been created to combat this disease. If you need to find psychological help, begin with your county Mental Health Association or ask your physician for a referral. Curing a child of anorexia nervosa can be a long, hard battle. You and your troubled child are going to need help to win it.

Bulimia

Bulimia is characterized as a binge-and-purge disorder. Bulimia victims frequently eat huge quantities of food and then quickly rid themselves of it, mostly by self-induced vomiting. They also tend to use or overuse laxatives and diuretics and to overexercise in an effort to rid themselves of any traces of food. Bulimics get caught in an obsessive pattern of overeating and voiding that is very hard on their bodies.

Purging has a long history as a method of weight control. The Romans routinely practiced it as part of their large banquets in order to be able to stuff themselves. The practice is not uncommon (though quite secret) today with people, usually women, who are trying to control their weight. Most seem to practice it on an occasional basis, however, not obsessively.

Bulimic girls (bulimia is relatively rare among boys) usually place themselves on strict diets in an effort to control what they see as self-indulgent and hideous fat. As a parent, you may not perceive a need for such a diet, but then many adolescent girls go through a phase in which they feel they must lose weight in order to be attractive. Food is often a comfort for bulimia victims, so after a period of strict dieting they break down and binge, which only reinforces their feelings of worthlessness: "If I can't even control the food I eat, I must be a terrible person," the bulimic imagines. Then she purges herself in an effort to regain control.

Signs to Look for

It is often difficult to recognize bulimia, since victims usually look perfectly normal. If you notice that large quantities of food have been disappearing, such as a gallon of ice cream in an afternoon, you might be tipped off. You might also hear your daughter vomiting frequently. Excessive weight loss is a good sign as well, but bulimics are usually not excessively thin. A bulimic's teeth may also begin to stain since gastric juices wear away the protective enamel.

Chances are also good that you will *not* notice such things. Bulimia is not a disorder that a victim wants anyone to know about. Bulimics often buy their own binge foods and then hide the wrappers. They also become quite adept at disguising the evidence of purging. It's hard to imagine being in a house with someone who vomits several times a day without being aware of it, but this is common.

If you suspect a problem, talk first to your daughter or son. Your child must recognize that there is a problem before you can get assistance. Once you've had the conversation, bring in professional help. First arrange for the child to have a complete physical. Then call your county Mental Health Association or family physician for the name of a qualified mental-health professional.

PART III
......
Food and Behavior

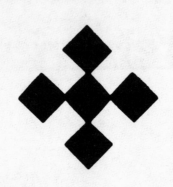

Introduction to Part III

• • • • • •

Food is a powerful medium. Not only does it affect our health, but it affects the way we feel. Certain foods can make us feel energetic; other foods can make us feel lethargic. If we don't eat enough, we may not be able to concentrate; and if we eat too much food—or the wrong kind—we may find ourselves carrying around added pounds and a self-image that could stand a boost.

A healthy attitude toward food helps us to be not only biologically well-nourished, but also socially well-nourished. Since so much of our socializing is centered around food, encouraging good table manners in your children will help them to feel confident in social situations. Exercise, too, is a great confidence-builder. Helping your child to enjoy physical activity will help him *feel* good, as well as *look* good. And what better way to build a positive self-image?

In this section, we'll discuss the varying effects different foods have on children's behavior, how diet and exercise affect self-esteem, and tips on encouraging good table manners, with advice from some of the best sources—parents themselves. We also include a special section on prevention of food-related hazards.

CHAPTER ELEVEN

······

How Does Diet Affect Children's Moods?

The way we feel about food has much to do with our "food mood," as does the food we eat. That's the emotional connection. There's also a physiological connection between food and the way we feel. Without *enough* food, or enough variety of foods, we become listless and unable to concentrate. Likewise, eating too heavily can slow us down, especially if we've eaten sugar-laden carbohydrates that temporarily boost our energy and then lead to a quick loss of energy. Certain substances in foods affect some people, too. Knowing when food is likely to affect mood and what foods in themselves can trigger negative reactions are the first steps in understanding the interaction between diet and behavior.

Timing

The body needs food about every four hours, except during sleep, when it slows down. This is one reason why breakfast is so important, especially for children. After seven or more hours without food, a child's body needs to refuel. Studies have been performed that show that children who have gone without breakfast have a shorter attention span and more difficulty concentrating than children who begin their days with breakfast. Not surprisingly, hungry children do poorly on tests. They also tend to be restless, no doubt because the hunger signals their bodies are sending out are distracting them from the tasks at hand.

It's not just a matter of when a child eats that matters, however. *What* he eats is critical as well. A breakfast of a sweet roll and nothing else is almost as likely to shorten his attention span by the middle of the morning—when the carbohydrates are no longer in his stomach—as no breakfast at all. This is because the quick energy provided by the sugar is used up and the body needs more fuel after an hour or two. If a glass of milk or other carbohydrate-protein mix is eaten in addition to the sweet roll, the body, which breaks down these elements more slowly, has longer-lasting fuel. And if he begins his day with a bowl of vitamin-enriched cereal, milk, and juice, he'll be even better armed to face the day. This is why a child needs a combination of foods: carbohydrates for quick energy and proteins and fats to provide long-term nutrients for the growth and repair of the body.

Particular Foods and Behavior

Does eliminating certain foods from children's diets help control children's behavior? Yes and no.

Caffeine

Certain substances, such as caffeine, can adversely affect a child's behavior when consumed in large quantities. Most adults know the effects of caffeine well. A cup or two of coffee or tea in the morning helps many people wake up and become alert. In the middle of the day, it can help you concentrate. However, when coffee is consumed in large quantities (four to eight cups a day or more), it can also raise the heart rate and other metabolic functions, producing "coffee jitters" and heart palpitations.

Children, too, are easily affected by caffeine. Few small children drink coffee, of course, but many drink colas and chocolate-based drinks, which can produce high levels of caffeine when consumed in quantity. These drinks contain much less caffeine ounce for ounce than coffee (30 to 36 milligrams per 6 ounces for cola, as opposed to 83 milligrams per 6 ounces of brewed coffee), but people drink 12-ounce servings of colas on the average, as opposed to 6-ounce servings of coffee. This means that the average serving of cola contains anywhere from 40 to 72 milligrams of caffeine, a hefty amount, especially for someone with a child's body weight. Experts estimate that a young child who drinks a can of cola gets the same kick as an adult who drinks four cups of coffee.

As is so often the case with issues of nutrition, the bottom line here is that moderation should be the rule. If a child has a well-balanced diet that includes a nutritious breakfast, a little caffeine probably won't alter his behavior. Large amounts of caffeine, however, should be avoided.

Food Additives

Food additives such as preservatives, food coloring, and sweeteners have been linked to changes in children's behavior, too. Some of these additives are found in nature (such as the sugar added to canned corn) or are synthetic copies of natural substances (such as ascorbic acid, which is used to preserve food; and carotene, the pigment found in carrots and other vegetables, which is used as food coloring). These additives actually add to the nutritional value of food and have not been shown to cause any undesirable effects. Additives such as the vitamins added to fortified milk and to grain products increase the nutritional value of food, too. Other synthetic additives, such as Aspartame (marketed under the brand names Nutrasweet or Equal), have been declared safe, but studies suggest that these additives may cause diarrhea or headaches in children who are sensitive to them. Many doctors recommend that children who are subject to migraine headaches avoid Aspartame entirely, since its ingestion has been linked to increased occurrence and severity of migraines. A small number of children *do* have allergies and, thus, negative reactions to other synthetic additives, but most children are not adversely affected by these products.

Sugar

There was a period in the 1970s when a limited amount of research seemed to indicate that children became hyperactive after eating sugar. At first, the theory made sense: A child would go to a birthday party, and the normally well-behaved but active youngster would go into a frenzy. At the end of the party, he would be irritable and weepy, sometimes having tantrums. All the sugar in the birthday cake and candy he ate—that must have done it! Initially, no one stopped to think that perhaps the excitement of the party and the gathering of high-spirited children might have had something to do with his extraordinary mood swings. Researchers also failed to take into account the fact that sugar has been used for centuries as a treat and pacifier.

Recently, however, studies have been made of the effects of sugar on children that draw different conclusions. It's been determined that sugar does give children a boost of extra energy—chemically, that is exactly what sucrose does—but it has not been found to be the cause of any negative behavior. In fact, recent research has shown that sugar may help improve children's attention spans slightly. Other studies have found that sugar makes some children sleepy rather than aggressive or hyperactive. And since few children are free from a craving for sweets, eliminating them from a child's diet is an unnecessary deprivation. Of course, refined sugar is not exactly a health food either. Like every other part of a child's diet, sugar consumption should be viewed in perspective. A moderate amount will not harm a child. Eating large quantities of processed, high-sugar foods, on the other hand, can leave a child too full to eat other, more nutritious foods. Eating fruit can satisfy the physical craving for sweets, while providing additional nutrition.

Some patients substitute honey-sweetened treats for sugar in the belief that honey is better for children than refined sugar, but this is not true. The body processes honey the same way it digests any other sugar; it doesn't know the difference. Honey *does* contain trace amounts of nutrients that refined sugar does not, but the amounts are so tiny that you would have to eat a tremendous amount of honey to achieve any real benefits. If you do prefer honey to sugar, there are two important considerations: (1) sweet, sticky, honey adheres to the teeth a little more firmly than do other sugars, making it somewhat more likely to cause tooth decay; and (2) honey contains bacteria that cannot be processed by an infant's immature digestive system. Thus, honey should *never* be given to children under one year of age.

Food and Children with Food Sensitivities

A small percentage of children are food sensitive or truly allergic. For most of these children, the primary reaction will be physical, with symptoms such as wheezing or hives. The discomfort caused by these physical reactions can, of course, alter a child's mood.

Some children's behavior, however, may be negatively affected by food or food additives. Before putting your child on a restrictive diet, it's important to work with a medical professional such as a nutritionist who is affiliated with a hospital. (Be suspicious of anyone who suggests a total switch to an unusual, nonbalanced diet; if you're feeling desperate about your child's behavior, there are those who are willing to take your money in exchange for the promise of a quick solution.) A qualified professional will ask you to record everything your child eats over a period of time and to note any unusual behavior. You will also be asked to note what activities your child is engaged in around the time that the behavior occurred. Very often, you'll find that other events and not food intake are the causes of unacceptable behavior.

If you do find that a food or additive is the suspected cause of misbehavior, you need to enlist your child's help, as well as the help of any other caregiver, in eliminating the offending food or additive from her diet. If the offending food is one that your child particularly likes, make it clear that she is not being punished when you withhold the food.

• •

Advice from Parents

Readers of *Sesame Street Magazine Parents' Guide* were asked:

Do you ever talk to your children about how their diet affects how they feel and act?

Their responses:

"Yes, we talk about the importance of eating right so they will have energy to play and read and do other things. My six-year-old is eager to play organized ball activities, so we insist on balanced meals to help him 'participate better.'

I also believe that we can help children develop healthy diet habits by the examples we set. At our house, we've greatly improved our diet recently, and I've found that the boys are more eager to try new foods, especially if my husband and I are more open to these same foods."

—Sally Hartley
Salix, IA

"We try to show them simple cause-and-effect relationships with food. For example, if my daughter says she is hungry in the mid-afternoon, I might tell her that it is because she did not eat all of her lunch. Or, if she is extremely thirsty, I might relate this to having eaten too many chips. This way, if she sees the cause and effect, she may make a more responsible decision about what and how much of something to eat the next time."

—Mary E. Kolb
East Greenbush, NY

"As toddlers, our children have always helped in the garden, making bread, and preparing supper. The simplest nutrition lessons, such as 'The sun and rain and good soil make the peas grow, and peas help make our bodies strong,' leave lasting impressions.

We have found that our children are apt to try many new foods if they help in picking or preparing them—and the questions they ask in the process are excellent nutrition-building stones. Our four- and seven-year-olds know why baked potatoes are healthier than French fries and that when their bodies are healthy and strong, they have enough energy to play and run, and grow and learn."

—Becky Perkins
Belle Plaine, MN

"Our children, ages six and five, already know that caffeine isn't good for them, and they look for it on food labels.

We were very cautious when our children were younger, trying to avoid high-sugar, caffeinated, and carbonated foods. Now they have taken over and would prefer to eat foods such as raisins and juice than candy and pop.

We make it a point to mention how tall they are growing from eating well and how bright and healthy their teeth have become."

—Tom and Laura McConnell
Jewett, OH

"Although I find serious talks about nutrition boring, I do encourage my children to create a colorful plate. If there are four colors, I declare their meal nutritionally balanced. For example: hamburgers—brown; mashed potatoes—white; celery—green; carrots—orange.

Also, I introduce a new food every two weeks or so. Everyone—even my husband who is a picky eater—must try two bites. John, my five-year-old, has become a fan of kiwi fruit, cantaloupe, and honeydew melon as a result of this practice."

—Cecilia Morelli
Sand Springs, OK

"The kids have been taught that too much candy, soda, or junk will give them a stomachache. I have also allowed them to learn through their own experience, and that has helped more than all the nagging I would ever have done. They remember and will say, 'I better not have a candy because I might get a tummyache like I did that day we went to the fair.' "

—Kitty Schlosser
Zamora, CA

"When we were on vacation, the children kept wanting various junk foods. I finally explained to them about 'animal fat' and how products that use animal fat for frying and as an ingredient are not good for us; they are high in cholesterol, they add extra pounds, etc. From that time on, every place we went, the kids would ask the waiter or waitress what their French fries were fried in, how the shrimp was prepared—on and on."

—Meg Hubbard
Littleton, CO

"At age four, my daughter already knows that too much sugar is undesirable. When we walk down the cereal aisle of our local grocery store and I shake my head 'no' at her request to try a particular cereal that she has seen on TV, she responds knowingly, 'Too much sugar, right, Mommy?' "

—Judith Sayre Grim
Littleton, CO

151

"I have talked with both my nine-year-old son and three-year-old daughter about products that contain caffeine and lots of sugar and why we avoid them.

My three-year-old is just starting to understand the difference between food that tastes good and food that is good for us, and that they're not always the same."

—Mrs. Drunette Roper
Hatfield, PA

"My girls Amanda, four-and-a-half, and Erika, two-and-a-half, are fruit and vegetable eaters. They'd rather have a carrot stick than a cookie. They know all about nutrition and how broccoli is better for them than cake.

I think my children are a lot more aware of how important good nutrition is than I was when I was growing up. Mainly because I'm probably more aware than my parents were."

—Karla Kinzie
Durand, MI

• •

CHAPTER TWELVE

······

Table-Time Behavior for Young Children

From the first time you and your baby make eye contact during feeding time, he is learning that food and eating are pleasurable, social activities. Parents expect very little in the way of manners during a child's first few months, and, in fact, a good loud burp after dinner is encouraged.

By the time a child reaches later babyhood and toddlerhood, he is learning the delights of squishing food with his fingers, flinging it across the room, and lathering it in his hair, all normal behaviors that he will soon outgrow—provided that he is neither reprimanded harshly nor encouraged to continue because he's learned that such behavior warrants lots of attention.

At what point, then, can parents consider instilling table manners in their children? The answer is: right from the start, though at the beginning this is best accomplished simply by setting the example you'd like your child to imitate, rather than by lecturing. Even a two-year-old who's making a mashed-potato mountain will notice if you say, ''Please pass the muffins,'' to your spouse and other children. Children who are encouraged to join pleasant dinner conversation rather than bear witness to dinnertime squabbles will be relaxed enough to absorb whatever table rules you consciously teach, too. And like other aspects of development, you can expect that children will learn social graces one step at a time, with regular backsliding being the rule rather than the exception. What can they learn, and when? While there are no set guidelines, parents can reasonably expect children to move from their natural, primitive eating habits to something resembling civilized behavior beginning at about age three. The following tips can help dissuade most children from continuing unacceptable mealtime behaviors:

Behavior	Tips
Food-flinging and/or mashing food into hair	• Give your child enough mealtime attention, so that these behaviors are not used to involve you in his feeding time. Try not to overreact, as these behaviors could become attention-getting devices.
Grabbing food	• Encourage the use of ''please'' and ''thank you.'' However, do *not* refuse your child his meal or snack for forgetting to ask for it nicely. No matter what the state of his manners, he has a right to eat.
Talking with food in mouth	• Gentle persuasion and a reminder that ''I can't understand what you're saying with your mouth full,'' will eventually get your message across.

Behavior	Tips
Blowing into drinks to form bubbles	• Kids love to see the great froth created by blowing bubbles. This activity also helps teach them control of their mouth muscles. However, it's not always a welcome behavior. You can encourage a child to refrain from bubble-blowing at the table, while allowing it at playtime with cups of plain water. (And for those old enough to know not to swallow the soapy froth, you can make bubble-blowing a great bathtime activity.)
Using fingers to eat	• Some foods, of course, are meant to be eaten with the fingers, but by the time a child is ready to enter kindergarten, he is ready to eat foods such as string beans, apple pie, and even French fries with a fork. One good way to encourage the use of utensils is to have special child-size spoons and forks avail-

Behavior	Tips
	able. No matter what utensils he's using, gentle encouragement and praise will lead him to opt for a fork.
Playing with food	• While younger children use food play to learn the basic properties of foods, children over the age of four or so can learn other ways to experiment. Helping out in the kitchen encourages continued curiosity about food while discouraging tabletime food play.
Dawdling over dinner	• Some people are just naturally slow eaters. If meals are stretching into marathons, however, you can simply encourage your child to eat as much as he can during your mealtime and allow him to eat again later if he's still hungry.
Speed eating	• Some people are naturally quick eaters, but eating too quickly can cause digestive problems and can lead to overeat-

Behavior	Tips
	ing. To help a child slow down, try serving various elements of the meal separately, stressing that he can have as much as he wants. Suggest that he chew slowly, many times, before swallowing.
Spilling drinks	• Until a child is at least six or seven, it's unreasonable to expect that milk or other beverages won't be spilled rather regularly. Young children simply don't have the depth perception to realize that a glass placed at the edge of the table is in direct line with their elbows.
Wiping hands and face with something other than napkin	• It's interesting that one attribute of men's clothing—three or four buttons at the base of a suit sleeve—is said to have originated by Napoleon who was trying to teach his soldiers table manners. (He designed uniforms with sharp buttons that would in-

Behavior	Tips
	jure anyone who wiped his face with his sleeve.) No such drastic measures are necessary to teach kids to use napkins. The best method is simply to have napkins available and to encourage their use.
Refuses to eat what you've prepared	• Getting your child interested in the food *preparation* can avert this problem. When it does arise, feed your child what he wants, if possible. It's never a good idea to either force a child to eat or to allow him to be hungry.
Belching	• Grade-schoolers, particularly, can become adept at making gross sounds at the dinner table and they really enjoy your negative reaction (in much the same way they enjoy your shock over using foul language). Try not to overreact, but make it clear that the behavior is unacceptable.

Restaurant Behavior

You never can tell what will happen when you take a child out to eat in a restaurant. One time he's perfectly behaved, a model of tidiness and good manners. The next time, he behaves like a whirling dervish. Older children, who have some experience using utensils and learning to wait for food to arrive, can be counted on to behave reasonably well, if they are not dealing with any particular upset in their lives. Babies, toddlers, and young preschoolers generally lack the experience to weather the particular frustrations of away-from-home eating. But this is the time they can start to learn. Parents can help by beginning with the understanding that young children don't have much of an attention span. Therefore, to be on the safe side, the best first-restaurant experience you can choose is the one that will get you in and out most quickly. (If there were no such thing as children, there would be no fast-food restaurants.) Fast-food places or restaurants where you can phone your order in ahead of time make the chances of completing a meal in relative peace much greater. Choosing a restaurant at which you know children are welcome makes things much easier, too. The atmosphere will be more relaxed, and there will be more tolerance for the high spirits of children. No matter what restaurant you choose, try to sit by a window where kids will have some distractions while waiting for the food to arrive. Bring crackers or other edibles with you to avoid letting hunger get the best of them while waiting for food to arrive. If paper placemats are available, offer some crayons to keep them entertained.

If a child *does* act up, one parent can and should remove the child from other diners' hearing range until the child regains some control. The next step, if composure isn't regained, is to leave the restaurant *calmly*. (If the food has already been ordered, ask for a "doggy bag.") Having a tantrum of your own won't solve the problem.

When Visiting

When dinner guests come to your house, you can expect a young child to forget some of the table manners he's learned, but at least you can find reasonable ways around any potential disruption. You can serve him earlier, allowing him to do most of his socializing away from the table, for instance. And you can make sure there's something on the menu that he'll like. Older children can be encouraged to show off for guests in a positive way by helping to serve hors d'oeuvres or by making placemats or printed menus.

When it's your family that's visiting, it can be more difficult to ensure a peaceful meal. It's not impossible, however. Just as when guests visit you at home, you can make sure a young child is not too hungry—and thus, cranky—at the table by feeding him a sandwich or side dish beforehand. Bring along some toys and other distractions if he's unable to sit at the table. It's helpful to keep in mind, too, that the point of most visits is not to eat but to socialize and to have fun. Focusing on your child's eating habits just now is not likely to accomplish the primary goal.

• •

Advice from Parents

Readers of *Sesame Street Magazine Parents' Guide* were asked:

What techniques do you use to encourage good table manners in your children?

Their responses:

"I point out how happy our children will make other people when they act appropriately and appreciatively. Manners are important in our family, and I *praise* the children when they use good manners."

—Michele Olson
Green Bay, WI

"We tell the children that people will treat them with more respect if they behave properly."

—Rich Mah
South Bend, IN

"We always use our behavior as an example. If the children start getting wild, we simply remove their plates and tell them they are finished. We usually give them one more chance to finish eating correctly."

—Amy Cohen
Columbia, MD

"We role-play table manners at play tea parties."

—Linda Johnson
Cleveland, AL

"The main problem we had regarding table manners was that our three-year-old son, Danny, was talking with a full mouth. He had a hard time remembering to close his mouth. Then I bought a *Golden Book* about manners. The funny characters in it kept his interest, plus taught him proper manners. It really worked!"

—Robyn Freiberger
Apple Valley, MN

"Once a month we have dinner at 'Chez Perkins.' Our dining table is transformed with a good tablecloth, our best china, lighted candles, and a printed menu. Each child gets a chance to be the 'wait-person' and help Chef Mom. Combed hair and clean faces start the meal and best manners are practiced. Because of the at-home practice, our kids are not intimidated by wedding receptions or the occasional fancy restaurant we splurge on. Friends and relatives compliment them on their manners when they visit. That, too, is a very effective reinforcer."

—Becky Perkins
Belle Plaine, MN

"We often ask Jenny, age nine, and David, age seven, to cook a meal. I'll do the shopping and help them if they need it. It's surprising how much is eaten and how respectfully when they themselves have cooked the meal!"

—Anna Hart
Alexandria, VA

"My favorite idea is to play 'restaurant' with my three children. I make construction-paper menus for each one, consisting of all the leftovers in the refrigerator. While I prepare, my 'customers' are busy grooming themselves. They know 'Polly's Restaurant' is top-of-the-line, and anyone with bad table manners or a poor attitude towards the meal will be asked to leave. We are all very polite and complimentary. The game ends after I total the bill and Josh, age nine, pays for everyone's dinner with play money from his wallet.''

—Polly Zwiebel
Maplewood, OH

''We feel that our children learn their table manners by example. And I feel this has been proven true. My husband and I are polite to each other; we say 'please' and 'thank you,' we do not talk with our mouths full, and we ask to be excused from the table. It takes no time at all for our kids to pick up on our manners and imitate us.

—Kitty Schlosser
Zamora, CA

''We try setting good examples and reminding the children what's acceptable at the table and what's not. When things get too out of hand, they are asked to leave the table. They may come back when they feel they are ready.''

—Mary Murray
Tinley Park, IL

''One way to help good manners along is that children should point out when *parents* omit such words as 'please' or 'thank you' by saying, 'Daddy, you didn't say please,' or 'Mommy is going to have a sore back because she's not sitting up straight.' Small reminders never hurt.''

—Theresa Chapman
Olean, NY

Readers of *Sesame Street Magazine Parents' Guide* were asked:

If you take your children to a restaurant, what do you do to keep them occupied during the wait and the meal?

Their responses:

"We eat out often with our two- and five-year-old boys and have since they were newborns. We frequent restaurants with large waiting areas where they can run around or with large grassy areas out front for stretching their legs before *and* after the meal. We always take a bag of Cheerios along to nibble on for these long waits. We also carry a couple of quiet little toys that they can play with before the food is served or after they have finished eating (since the kids usually finish before we do and need something to keep them occupied while *we* eat). I also always carry four to six crayons in a Ziploc bag in my purse so the kids can draw on paper placemats."

—Linda Anicich
Placentia, CA

"For starters, we only take them to restaurants that accommodate children. Mexican and Chinese are good because there are chips or noodles on the table while you're waiting for your food. Salad bars are great because we can give them a small plate of goodies while we wait."

—Amy Cohen
Columbia, MD

"During the meal my kids usually finish first. So my husband and I order them a little dish of ice cream to keep them busy while we enjoy the rest of our meal."

—Sandy Butze
Riverside, CA

"Enjoyable conversation is one reason people go to restaurants, so we wanted to encourage and develop good conversational skills as well as proper restaurant etiquette with our children. When we take our girls (ages three and five) to a restaurant, we take along several photographs that usually focus on a specific topic, such as the children's baby pictures, our trip to Disneyland, or their grandparents. The photos help generate conversation, and the girls never seem to get tired of looking at the photos and hearing stories about when they were small. They also share their impressions. A picture is indeed worth a thousand words."

—Jonelle Whitney
Manchester, MO

"We don't eat out often; when we do, it's usually at a place where children are welcome. We look for places that have entertainment for children, such as balloons, crayons, games on placemats, etc."

—Margie Weissgerber
Orlando, FL

"While waiting for our meal, we point out things of interest, such as paintings on the wall, floral arrangements (our son loves flowers), or people we might know. I always have paper and a pen with me so that he can draw pictures.

During the meal we include him in our conversation as much as possible.''

—Diane Hanton
Ellis Grove, IL

''We bring along books to look at or color in—along with crayons or markers. We also play the game 'Twenty questions' on a lower level—we say, 'I'm thinking of something that's _____' and describe an object in the room. Each child takes a turn, and soon the food has come and we can eat.''

—Rich Mah
South Bend, IN

''Discussing the menu and letting our child decide among predetermined choices keeps her involved. Also, if she orders for herself, its a much more interesting event.''

—Laura Skaggs
Louisville, KY

''Many parents put their tots into high chairs immediately upon being seated, but I allow mine to sit in a regular chair or booth until the food is actually served. Somehow, the shorter time spent in a high chair improves his behavior.''

—Cecilia Morelli
Sand Springs, OK

''Save all your 'stories' for at the restaurant instead of in the car on the way to the restaurant.''

—Gaye L. Sanders
Hastings, MI

"After we order, we often take our eighteen-month-old for a walk or stroll around the restaurant or lobby until the food arrives. This helps to alleviate his restlessness."

—P. Guerrieri
Virginia Beach, VA

"I have found that asking to keep a menu during the waiting period passes the time quickly. I read everything on the menu, taking time to answer their questions ('What's an appetizer? How do you eat a lobster?') and explain terms such as *à la mode*. This puts the kids in an eating mood and they remain intent until the meal arrives."

—Polly Jo Zwiebel
Maplewood, OH

"Here are some things that work when we eat out with our five-year-old and two-year-old:

- Go early enough (if possible) to avoid the rush—you get waited on and served faster.

- Some restaurants serve children from glasses that are too big for them to handle so I bring plastic cups with lids from home.

- When you order, ask the waiter or waitress to bring more napkins ahead of time."

—Mary Murray
Tinley Park, IL

● ●

CHAPTER THIRTEEN

• • • • • •

Body Types, Body Weight, and Self-Image

There are many different body types, and our individual body type is with us from the day we are born. Some people are long and lean; others are short and squat; others are a combination of the two. Our basic body configurations are determined by genetics, not by diet or exercise. Tall, angular parents are more likely to have tall, angular children, just as broad, chunky parents are more likely to produce chunky kids.

In addition to genes, each individual's metabolism (the way the body uses fuel) has a lot to do with determining body shape. Even people who look similar may use the fuel in their bodies in very different ways. Some people burn more calories using less food than others. One person at rest can be burning calories while another is storing the calories as fat. Sometimes you can spot the real calorie-burners by their constant fidgeting, but that is not always the case. In some instances, energy is burned when a person is under emotional stress.

A really efficient body will burn calories slowly, storing more for later use. Thus, an overweight person's system may actually work more efficiently than a thin person's, which requires greater amounts of fuel. Unlike your genetic makeup, your metabolism *can* be changed; you can raise the speed at which your body burns calories through aerobic exercise, which burns fat. However, unless you continue to be more active, your basal metabolic rate will return to normal, even if normal for you is very slow indeed.

Do children with different body types need different diets? Sometimes yes, sometimes no. We all know families whose members all seem to be constantly thin and constantly eating. They eat huge meals and snack on gallons of ice cream, but still they stay thin, so much so that the children may appear undernourished. We all know families in which the opposite is true, too, with everyone overweight and on a perpetual diet. In some families, only one or two members have a predisposition one way or another.

Children at either extreme often need special diets. A child who is more than 15 percent below what's recommended for her age and build needs extra food, while one who is more than 15 percent over the recommended weight may need a reduced-calorie diet and an increase in activity. A child who is a little chubby or one who is somewhat thin probably doesn't need a special diet; she may just need to wait six months. Many chunky boys and girls slim down when they start to add inches to their height. Thin children, too, tend to broaden as they enter adolescence.

Before helping your overweight or underweight child to design a new diet, there are two other important things parents can do: (1) teach the basics of sound nutrition, primarily by example; and (2) instill self-esteem in your child so that she will feel good about the body she has.

Body Weight and Self-Image

As we think back to our own childhoods, we can all remember the kids in class who stood out: the smartest boy and girl, the most athletic, the most artistic, the prettiest, the handsomest, the funniest. These were the kids we admired and wanted to be like. Then there were those at the other end of the spectrum, the ones we feared we were or might become: the clumsiest, the least popular, the skinniest, the fattest.

Our notions of what is attractive and desirable begin very early, and, with the help of the media, we are all led to believe that fat is unattractive and that a fat person is somehow morally deficient or at the very least, simply lazy. Vicki Lansky, in her book *Fat-Proofing Your Children,* discusses the results of a study published in *Parents* magazine which measured the perceptions of adults and children regarding overweight children. When the respondents were asked to rate the attractiveness of a group of children, overweight children in the sample were ranked as less appealing than those confined to wheelchairs, those with a facial disfigurement, and those with limbs missing.

Of all traits, body weight is the one that people tend to judge most because it is a characteristic that is thought to be entirely within an individual's control. When a child walks down the street, no one can tell that she's regional spelling champ or an undefeated badminton player. Everyone knows what she looks like, though, even from a distance.

Girls are particularly sensitive about their shape and weight. During the teen years, body shape can create an emotional hardship for many. Teens' growth spurts make them grow up and out. Boys grow tall and broad of shoulder, increasing their muscle and bone mass. Girls grow tall and broad of hip, increasing their fat content. This is normal, one of the results of hormonal activity. In girls, the female hormone estrogen goes to work promoting and maintaining fat to prepare the body for bearing children. In boys, the male hormone testosterone is acting to build muscles and burn fat.

All of these changes are going on at a time when a child's self-image is of paramount importance. For children who have never had a weight problem, puberty can be hard enough. For those who have been heavy since they were young, or who have recently put on weight, the extra pounds can compound the problems of growing up. Likewise, being too thin can cause growing teens to think of themselves as less-than-ideal specimens.

Since having a good self-image is the key to dealing with any of life's challenges, including maintaining optimum body weight, teaching a child to feel good about her body is essential to her emotional and physical well-being. Most child-development experts agree that the starting point for building a child's self-esteem is her parents' own degree of self-esteem. In other words, if you like yourself, you are more likely to be confident with your children and to communicate your confidence in them. Parents who accept their children as they are are in a better position to help their children deal with any external (or internal) assaults on their self-esteem. Children need to know that being overweight or underweight has no bearing on the kind of people they are inside, what values they hold, and how successful they can be. Coincidentally, a child who feels good about herself is much more likely to follow a somewhat restricted diet because she values herself enough. She also trusts her own ability to succeed on a diet.

• •
Advice from Parents

Readers of *Sesame Street Magazine Parents' Guide* were asked:

What approaches do you use to help your children develop positive self-images and feel good about their bodies?

Their responses:

"We are consistent in praising our children's appearance. For instance, when our two-year-old puts on her Sunday dress, I tell her how pretty she looks and to go show Daddy. Daddy then compliments her and sends her to look in the mirror and admire herself.

We've tried to stress the connection between good foods and healthy bodies by talking about nutrition and vitamins and what each one does to help the body. The kids also like to exercise with Mom, and we talk about how everybody is special and, as long as you're healthy, you've got something to work with."

—Donnita Nesbit Fisher
Dallas, TX

"Sometimes my daughter gets discouraged about being small or having to wear glasses. My husband and I try to give her extra attention during those times and reassure her how much we love her just the way she is."

—Mary Murray
Tinley Park, IL

"I encourage my three-year-old daughter to run, jump, climb, explore—to test her limits. I don't think anything builds confidence like success."

—Laura Skaggs
Louisville, KY

"Even though my four-year-old son isn't always 'picture perfect,' I find that a little praise from Mom, such as 'Oh, what a handsome boy!' or 'What a great job you did combing your hair!' gets a big, proud smile from him and encourages him to do even better the next time he's dressing."

—Valeria Infantino
Pittston, PA

"I always use positive phrases to describe my son's actions. For example, 'You're a good jumper, aren't you,' or 'You really are learning how to share.' I never say, 'You're bad' or say anything to make him think that badness is inherent in his personality.'

—Amy Cohen
Columbia, MD

"We tell our four-year-old how beautiful she is all the time. We point out her best features by telling her all the wonderful things she inherited from both sides of the family—like her grandpa's eyes, her daddy's ears, her grandma's nose, her mommy's dimples, and her aunt's hair. It makes her feel good to know that she was made up of so many wonderful people."

—Sandy Butze
Riverside, CA

"I use correct body names and explain clearly the functions of each part. I try to stress the relationship of good health habits and strong bodies. Most of all, my husband and I both maintain a positive self-image so that our life reflects good nutrition, exercise, moderation, and above all else, *respect* for each other's bodies."

—Orissa Barbour
Naples, NY

"If I ever notice our children looking at their reflection, I try to mention something nice about them, such as, 'That sure is a kind little girl,' or 'He sure seems like a boy who is willing to share with others.' "

—Tom and Laura McConnell
Jewett, OH

"We have tried to let our son know that all different kinds of foods are important for good growth and that too much of anything isn't good.

Of course, we also make a point of praising him for all the things he does well—whether it's cleaning up after himself or jumping high. When he has done something inappropriate, we say, 'That was bad' or 'wrong' but *never* that he is bad. We have never used the words 'stupid' or 'dumb' or anything similar. We tell him we love him, that we are proud of him, that he is special."

—Margie Weissgerber
Orlando, FL

"I stress the importance of good eating habits and exercise. I go for mile walks with them every day. We also ride bikes and like to swim."

—Gaye L. Sanders
Hastings, MI

"My five-year-old son is just starting to be interested in grooming. He wets his little brush, stands in front of the mirror, and fixes his hair. I always make a fuss and tell him how handsome he is and what a big boy he's getting to be. Now, he insists on getting dressed by himself with little or no help. I feel that positive praise is essential, and with ongoing flattery, he will build self-esteem.

Hygiene is very important at this time. After he brushes his teeth, I feel it is essential to praise the appearance of his smile and how handsome or cute he looks. After all, these are lifetime habits, and we want them to endure as something that brings self-esteem, not as a chore."

—Kathleen L. Tansey
West Chester, PA

"John and I teach our four-year-old daughter Melody good grooming habits. We compliment her often and tell her the differences when she asks about a boy's body. We teach her how God made her and of his loving creativity in making her body, so she knows that she is loved."

—Sara Rytkonen
Eielson AFB, AK

"Taking time to comment on each child's growth is a great image-builder. My husband and I kiddingly mourn, 'Look, everybody. We used to have a little tiny baby Jeremy and now all we have is this big boy who's smart and eats as much as Mom and runs faster than Dad.' The kids love the attention."

—Polly Jo Zwiebel
Maplewood, OH

• •

CHAPTER FOURTEEN

......

Helping Children Take Charge of Their Own Diets

Teaching a child respect for himself begins with respecting him. This means allowing him to make his own decisions on as many fronts as possible, including food. Involving your child in nutrition education is a good method of showing him that you respect his good sense. Once he understands which foods are best for him, he should be involved in the decisions about what to eat. After all, it is his body, and what goes into it is ultimately his choice, not his parents' choice.

If you think that your child needs a special diet, start by taking him for a complete physical examination to a sympathetic health-care worker, perhaps a nutritionist who specializes in treating children. You may also want to consider enlisting the aid of an outside role model, such as a favorite teacher, scout leader, or family friend, to encourage the child to get his weight under control. (Children who resist the efforts of their parents may respond more favorably to a sympathetic outsider.)

Feeding the Overweight Child

Most overweight children don't need diets or special diet foods; they just need to learn to eat fewer high-calorie, low-nutrient-value foods and, most important, they need to exercise a little more.

When you are considering the best ways to feed an overweight child, take time to examine your family's diet as a whole. Do you serve a good variety of foods? Are fruits and vegetables important for snacks as well as meals? Do you keep fatty snacks and sodas (both the sugary and the diet kind) around the house, or do you encourage—especially by example—the eating of fruit, vegetables, plain crackers, and other nutritious snacks? Do you cook with a lot of fat and sugar? Do you eat chicken and fish more than beef and pork, and do you trim them of fat before cooking? This may be the time to reevaluate how you cook and eat. The whole family can benefit from a diet in which the consumption of fats and simple carbohydrates, such as cookies and chips, is lowered and consumption of complex carbohydrates, such as fruit, vegetables, bread, and grain, is increased. Make everyone's portion sizes a little smaller and don't automatically offer seconds. (You might want to keep serving dishes out of sight.) It's a lot easier for the overweight child to eat the right things when his whole family does.

Bake or broil foods instead of frying them, and cut down on the amount of fats used to season foods, too. A teaspoon of butter or margarine served on steamed vegetables will probably satisfy everyone as much as a tablespoon or more. They might even like a squeeze of lemon juice, instead. Low-calorie popcorn served without butter can be just as pleasing to most people as fried potato or corn chips—especially if it's the only thing available.

Again, don't treat an overweight child differently from the rest of the family. For instance, don't ever forbid him to eat high-calorie foods while allowing others in the family to do so. Don't nag him about his eating habits or his weight. Nagging will only make him resentful and guilty. It will *not* make him thin.

The Need for Exercise

Many overweight children do not eat more than their average-weight peers. Some even eat less. More important than the amount of food eaten is the fact that overweight children tend to be much less physically active than their leaner friends. Children of normal weight usually balance their food needs with their energy expenditure. The more they move around, the more they eat and vice versa. Chubbier children generally eat the same amount regardless of whether they have exercised or not. They don't consume more calories than other children; they just burn fewer.

Overweight kids have a chicken-and-egg problem when it comes to exercise: Because of their excess weight, it's uncomfortable, and perhaps embarrassing, to exercise, so they abstain from movement and keep gaining weight, which makes exercise even less appealing.

One of the keys to successful weight control for anyone, adult or child, is getting exercise on a regular basis. We hear a great deal about how unfit America's youngsters are, even in the middle of the current exercise boom. While more and more parents today are huffing and puffing through their routines, their kids are home watching TV. In any case, kids need exercise like everyone else, and a child with a weight problem needs it most. "Exercise," of course, is not limited to push-ups and aerobic dancing, although both activities can be handled by most children. The best physical activities for children, however, are the kind that encourage interaction among playmates—such as biking, running, and climbing—thus building social skills along with muscles.

One of the best things parents can do for all of their kids is to make exercise a regular part of their lives from an early age. Emphasize how good exercise makes *you* feel (not how good it makes you look). With young children, a playful exercise program can start with stretches with Mom or Dad and move walking, jogging, and swimming together. Arrange family outings that revolve around activity. As kids get older, take them bowling, horseback riding, or roller skating. Go for hikes in the country or fly kites on the beach. Have fun.

Whatever the weight status of your child is, you can help him cope with it. Ultimately, for all children's weight problems the prescription is the same: a balanced diet of good food, exercise—and affection.

Special Section: Prevention of Food-Related Hazards

• • • • • •

Just when you can stop worrying about whether your infant will ever sleep through the night, he starts crawling around and putting strange things in his mouth, things he can choke on as well as those that can poison him.

One of the best ways to prepare for ingestion-related emergencies is to take a first-aid or CPR (cardiopulmonary resuscitation) course *before* you need it. The American Red Cross, local hospitals, and many other organizations nationwide offer courses throughout the year for free or for a nominal fee. Such courses teach proper resuscitation methods and give you the opportunity to practice the techniques under professional guidance and without the pressure of an emergency situation. There are often special programs aimed at showing parents how to cope with specific infant- and child-related emergencies. Another measure you can take *before* an emergency arises is to post the phone number of your local poison-control center and paramedic emergency squad so that they're immediately available when needed. It is also important to have a fresh bottle of syrup of ipecac on hand. This substance induces vomiting, which is the first-aid remedy for certain forms of poisoning.

Choking

Infants sometimes choke for no apparent reason when they're being breast- or bottle-fed. When an infant becomes flooded by a sudden rush of milk, he can choke. He will usually cough, sputter, and cry, probably scaring both his parents and himself. When this happens, place the baby in a sitting position and let him cough for a while before you start feeding again. If you are breast-feeding, you may be able to prevent the problem by expressing a little milk by hand before you offer your breast to the baby. Bottle-fed babies can be helped by propping them in a position closer to sitting than to lying down during feedings.

Until all his teeth are in and his chewing abilities are well established, a toddler is likely to swallow some foods whole, which can cause choking. This is particularly dangerous because a young child's air passage is narrow, and his mechanism for coughing up obstructing foods is underdeveloped. Certain hard foods, such as raw carrot sticks, hot dogs, peanuts, popcorn nuts, olives, and grapes should be avoided in order to lessen the chance of choking in young children. Good chewing skills are usually developed by about the age of three or four.

To cut down on the number of near-choking incidents in your home:

- Cut up all toddlers' solid food into small pieces.

- Teach children the habit of chewing food thoroughly.

- Supervise young children during meals and snacks.

- Don't allow a child to eat or drink while lying down.

- Teach children not to toss food into their mouths or pour candies into an upturned mouth.

- Check toys frequently for loose or broken pieces that could create a potential hazard.

- Baby- and toddler-proof your home, removing from reach all small-sized ingestible hazards such as buttons, coins, erasers, beads and other jewelry, and bottle caps.

Poisoning

It's a jungle out there—at least as viewed through the eyes of a curious toddler. When children begin exploring the world on their own, everything they can touch belongs to them, and everything they own can be swallowed.

The best way to see what is in reach of your locomoting child is to get down to his height and tour the house yourself, perhaps even following him around to see what attracts his eye. Things look different from floor level, and you will probably notice things that you've never seen before. Anything dangerous should be picked up and placed out of reach. It's important, too, to realize that children are adept at opening drawers and cabinets. Rather than banishing a child from all low cupboards, fill them instead with items that are safe playthings, such as pots and pans, and remove *all* cleaning products and other ingestibles from a child's reach.

Make sure all medicines are in bottles with childproof caps, too. Be aware, however, that children have been known to open even "childproof" caps with ease. Therefore, all medicines should be well out of the reach of children, in a high closet or a locked cabinet. The same is true

of perfumes, bathing products, and any gardening chemicals. House and garden plants can be poisonous, too, and
are best kept well beyond the reach of children.

Tainted food and undercooked or raw eggs can cause
poisoning, too, and adults are equally susceptible to this
hazard. The following steps can be taken to avoid food
poisoning in your home:

- Never serve raw or undercooked eggs.
- Wash your hands thoroughly after handling raw or un-
dercooked meats.
- Wash cutting boards and utensils that have been in con-
tact with meat thoroughly with soap and hot water.
Avoid wooden cutting boards altogether since any cracks
can make it impossible to clean them properly.
- Do not refreeze raw frozen foods.
- Teach children to wash their hands before and after eat-
ing.

First Aid for Poisoning

No matter how hard you've tried to protect your child, one
day he might swallow something poisonous. Here's what
to do:

If Poison Has Been Ingested:

1. In the event that poison has been swallowed, try to find
out what has been taken and call the nearest poison-
control center, physician, hospital, or rescue squad.
*These numbers should be posted near every phone in your
home.*
2. Do *not* induce vomiting, unless advised to do so or unless you're *sure* that the ingested poison should be ex-

pelled. (Some caustic poisons cause additional damage on their way up.)

3. If inducing vomiting is called for, administer the recommended dosage of syrup of ipecac, a drug that should be in every family's medicine chest and replaced frequently to ensure its freshness.

4. Take the child to a medical facility. Carry the complete package, container, or remnants of whatever the child has ingested. Also take along a pan or tray to collect any vomit. The medical personnel may need to examine it.

If Poison Has Been Inhaled

1. If the child has inhaled something toxic, take him into the fresh air immediately.

2. If the child is not breathing, begin mouth-to-mouth breathing.

3. Call the rescue squad.

Pica

The routine eating of such things as dirt, sand, grass, plaster, paint, paper clips, and even animal feces is a problem among some children. The disorder is called *pica*, from the Greek word for "magpie," a bird known for its scavenging.

Most common among toddlers, pica may be a signal of iron-deficiency anemia or lack of another mineral or vitamin, so your first reaction to this kind of behavior should be to take your child to a doctor for a check-up to determine if such a deficiency exists. If paint or dirt has been eaten in any large quantity, over an extended period, the child may also have been exposed to excessive levels of lead and thus to lead poisoning, which can have serious consequences to his physical and mental growth.

It's possible, however, that the problem is not physical but emotional. One of the reasons that pica occurs most often during toddlerhood is that children of that age are beginning to demand an enormous amount of attention, and eating dirt is sometimes the best way they know to get it. Pica can also be the result of a problem between child and parent or a child's reaction to stresses within the family.

It's important to handle pica calmly. If a parent displays anger or fear when faced with a child eating dirt or other nonfood substances, the child's craving for attention may be fulfilled, thus reinforcing the behavior. A better method is to try to offer a distraction while stating calmly and matter-of-factly that eating dirt (or whatever) is not allowed. Sometimes children need to revert a little in their behavior while getting over this problem. Some parents find that allowing the child to play more with his food at mealtime helps, as does reintroducing the use of a pacifier.

Afterword:
Putting It All Together

• • • • • •

All parents want what's best for their children—a good education, happiness, success, health. If we had our way, all our kids would be happy and healthy all the time. Understandably enough, we want to do everything in our power to make that ideal scenario a reality, and that includes making sure that our children eat the kinds of foods that will make them grow healthy, fit, and strong.

In this guide, we have tried to give you a push in that direction, arming you with the most up-to-date information about your growing child's nutritional needs and offering practical advice about how best to fulfill these needs. We hope we've given you some comfort as well. If you are like most parents, you are relieved to know that other parents are in the same boat—that yours is not the only toddler on the planet who refuses to eat anything green, for instance. Sharing your experiences can be a great help, too.

Good nutrition is vitally important to your child's health, and that is a serious business, indeed. But this doesn't mean that when you sit down to your family meals, you should lose your sense of humor. No matter what the issue is, a sense of humor is one of a parent's most valuable assets. So pass the vegetables and keep smiling!

Resources

......

Organizations

American Anorexia/Bulimia Association, 133 Cedar Lane, Teaneck, NJ 07666. (201) 836–1800

This is an information and referral service for people with eating disorders and their parents. It offers counseling and organizes self-help groups in Virginia, Pennsylvania, Florida, New York, and New Jersey. Additionally, it has a nationwide directory of therapists and hospital treatment centers and a newsletter published five times a year.

ANAD—National Association of Anorexia Nervosa and Associated Disorders, Box 7, Highland Park, IL 60035. (312) 831–3438 *(hotline number)*

This nonprofit international association is dedicated to alleviating and preventing the problems of eating disorders. It sponsors a broad public-education program to prevent eating disorders and has compiled the largest and most complete research on this topic in the nation.

ANAD's services include a national hotline (312–831–3438), staffed by people who have experienced eating disorders; free self-help support groups in forty-five states and five foreign countries; and a quarterly newsletter.

Children's Better Health Institute, 1100 Waterway Boulevard, P.O. Box 567, Indianapolis, IN 46206. (317) 636–8881

This organization, which is part of the Benjamin Franklin Literary and Medical Society, publishes material designed to help children of preschool through elementary school levels learn about health, nutrition, safety, and exercise, and provides parents with medical information concerning infants and children.

Publications include *Children's Health Connection, Child Life, Children's Digest, Health Explorer,* and *Humpty Dumpty.*

Children's Foundation, 815 15th Street NW, Suite 928, Washington, DC 20005. (202) 347–3300

This is a national advocacy organization that provides a voice for children and their families on issues of critical concern on both the national and local levels. Its major concerns are child care—especially family day care—and the problems created by the growing feminization of poverty.

Publications include a newsletter—*The National Family Day Care Bulletin*—and the *Factsheet on Child Care Food Program in Family Day Care Homes.*

Food and Nutrition Service, U.S. Department of Agriculture, 3101 Park Center Drive, Room 819, Alexandria, VA 22302. (703) 756–3281

This agency of the federal government runs programs designed to stop people from being hungry. It provides food stamps to eligible participants, a child-care food program, and vouchers for pregnant women to obtain special food packages, tailored to their nutritional needs, from their local grocery store. For more information on these programs, contact your local welfare office.

Publications available include *How WIC Helps—Eating for You and Your Baby, Building a Better Diet,* and *Make Your Food Dollars Count.*

Formula (Infants), P.O. Box 39051, Washington, DC 20016. (203) 527–7171

This organization is concerned with ensuring the safety and nutritional completeness of all infant formulas. By gathering data from parents whose children have suffered learning disabilities, gross motor dysfunction, seizures, and other symptoms as a result of having been fed Neo-Mull or Cho-Free (infant formulas manufactured without chloride by the Syntex Corporation), it has helped affected children receive proper medical attention. *Formula* serves as an information center and communication link for concerned parents.

Gesell Institute of Human Development, 310 Prospect Street, New Haven, CT 06511. (203) 777–3481 (Frani Pollack, Nutritionist)

This is a private, nonprofit research organization founded by Dr. Arnold Gesell in 1911. Its work deals with child growth and development, child behavior, child psychology, and developmental assessment.

The institute offers individual counseling on matters related to nutrition and eating disorders. For those who do not live locally, the institute will answer questions over the phone.

National Center for Education in Maternal and Child Health (NCEMCH), 38th & R Streets NW, Washington, DC 20057. (202) 625–8400

This organization provides information on such topics as human genetics, nutrition, sudden-infant-death syndrome, nursing, child health, maternal health, and prevention of disease and illness.

NCEMCH services, which are free, include the identification, listing, and dissemination of single copies of a wide variety of government publications in these areas. The *Publications List,* available on request, is a valuable annotated list of government documents on child and maternal health.

Nutrition—Adult Titles

Better Homes and Gardens. *Healthy Foods for Hungry Kids.* Des Moines, IA: Meredith, 1987.

Easy-to-follow recipes, with enticing color photographs. Nutritious and delicious selections. Available in hardcover and paperback.

Better Homes and Gardens. *Kids' Lunches.* Des Moines, IA: Meredith, 1986.

Delicious, nutritious, for home, on the go, and school. Paperback.

Brink, Jan, and Melinda Ramm. *S.N.A.C.K.S. (Speedy, Nutritious and Cheap Kids' Snacks).* New York: New American Library, 1984.

Like the title says. Available in hardcover and paperback.

Brody, Jane. *Jane Brody's Good Food Book: Living the High-Carbohydrate Way.* New York: W.W. Norton, 1985.

A step-by-step guidebook to healthful eating for the entire family. Ms. Brody inspires readers toward good nutrition with her careful and well-researched analysis of what good nutrition is. The detailed suggestions she offers on how to incorporate this information into your own family's regime are sensible and invitingly practical. More than 350 recipes. Available in hardcover and paperback.

Brody, Jane. *Jane Brody's Nutrition Book: A Lifetime Guide to Good Eating for Better Health and Weight Control by the Personal Health Columnist of* The New York Times. New York: W.W. Norton, 1985.

Although published more than seven years ago, this remains one of the best books of its kind, with clear and detailed explanations, sound advice, recipes, and enough information to help you make intelligent decisions about your family's diet. Includes sections on nutrition relating to pregnancy, babies, breast-feeding, children and junk food, adolescents, athletes, and overweight and underweight conditions. Hardcover. Also available in paperback from Bantam.

Caplan, Frank, ed. *The Parenting Advisor,* by the Princeton Parenting Center for Infancy. New York: Anchor/Doubleday, 1978.

In this overall guide for parents there is a chapter on feeding and nutrition which discusses breast-feeding versus bottle-feeding, weaning, making your own baby food, self-feeding, and overfeeding. Paperback.

Carper, Jean. *Jean Carper's Total Nutrition Guide.* New York: Bantam, 1987.

A comprehensive analysis of the vital nutrients in more than 2,500 foods. Includes specific nutritional guidelines for infants, children, and pregnant women; and charts, tables, and chapters with detailed discussions of particular nutrients: what they do, where to find them, and how to use them for optimum health benefits. Paperback.

Cohen, Mindy, M.A., and Louis Abramson. *Thin Kids: The Proven, Healthy, Sensible Weight-Loss Program for Children.* New York: Beaufort, 1985.

Based on a program designed to treat kids as they are, not as miniature adults. Covers self-image, exercise, strategies for success, menus, and recipes. Low-key approach. Available in hardcover and paperback.

Connor, Sonja L., M.S., R.D., and William E. Connor, M.D. *The New American Diet.* New York: Simon & Schuster, 1986.
Based on the five-year Family Heart Study sponsored by the National Institutes of Health and supervised by the authors, the New American Diet is a high-carbohydrate, low-fat diet that relies on gradual food substitutions in three phases over a period of three years. Sample menus, recipes, useful tips, and clear explanations are included in this sensible diet for the entire family. Hardcover.

Coyle, Rena with Patricia Messing, nutritionist. *Baby Let's Eat.* New York: Workman, 1987.
Information on how to adapt wholesome family meals for babies plus complete nutritional guidelines for children six months to three years, weekly menus for toddlers and special advice for feeding overweight children. Paperback.

Dodson, Fitzhugh, Ph.D., and Ann Alexander, M.D. *Your Child: Birth to Age 6.* New York: Simon & Schuster, 1986.
This overall guide to child development, discipline, and health care includes specific chapters on nutrition from pregnancy and breast-feeding through infancy, toddlerhood, and adolescence. Paperback.

Eisenberg, Arlene and Heidi Eisenberg Murkoff and Sandee Eisenberg Hathaway, R.N. *What to Eat When You're Expecting.* New York: Workman, 1986.
Practical and reassuring manual of nutrition for pregnant women. Paperback.

Epstein, Leonard H., Ph.D. and Sally Squires, M.S. *The Stoplight Diet for Children (An Eight-Week Program for Parents and Children.* Boston: Little, Brown, 1987.
Reasonable approach for parents to use to help overweight children lose and maintain weight loss. Practical and compassionate.

Finsand, Mary Jane. *Cooking for the Hyperactive Child*. San Diego: Oak Tree.

Recipes, plus list of food products which meet standards for hyperactive diet. Available in hardcover and paperback.

Hartbarger, Janie Coulter, and Neil J. Hartbarger. *Eating for the Eighties: A Complete Guide to Vegetarian Nutrition*. Philadelphia: Saunders/Holt, 1986.

Chapters on eating during pregnancy and guidelines for feeding babies and children. Available in hardcover and paperback.

Lambert-Lagace, Louise. *Feeding Your Child (From Infancy to Six Years Old)*. Revised edition. New York: Beaufort, 1983.

Menus, recipes, advice, and practical tips on healthful eating, prenatal through age six, by noted Canadian nutritionist. Paperback.

Lansky, Vicki. *Fat-Proofing Your Children . . . (So That They Never Become Diet-Addicted Adults)*. New York: Bantam, 1988.

A commonsense, practical way to establish lifelong health patterns for eating enough of the right foods for the right reasons to avoid problems in later life. Includes sections on teen eating disorders. Hardcover.

Lansky, Vicki. *Feed Me I'm Yours*. New York: Bantam, 1981.

How to get infants off to a nutritious head start. Recipes and advice. Paperback.

Lansky, Vicki. *The Taming of the C.A.N.D.Y.* Monster (*Continuously Advertised, Nutritionally Deficient, Yummies!): How to Get Your Kids to Eat Less Sugary, Salty Junk Foods . . . Without Sacrificing Convenience or Good Taste*. New York: Bantam, 1982.

Practical advice, tips, and more than 200 recipes. Paperback.

Leach, Penelope. *Your Baby and Child: From Birth to Age Five*. New York: Knopf, 1979.

Special sections on nutrition are arranged under chapters for each specific age grouping. Reassuring, specific advice. Available in hardcover and paperback.

Levenkron, Steven. *Treating and Overcoming Anorexia Nervosa*. New York: Charles Scribner's, 1982.

RESOURCES

A compelling, comprehensive, jargon-free look at anorexia: the patient, the family, the pathology, and the treatment, by the author of *The Best Little Girl in the World*. Available in hardcover and paperback.

Meyer, Tamara. *Help Your Child Build a Healthy Body: A New Exercise and Massage Program for the First Five Formative Years*. New York: Crown, 1984.
Beginning chapters explain the value of massage and exercise; later chapters offer detailed instructions, with photographs. Available in hardcover and paperback.

Natow, Annette, and Jo-Ann Heslin. *No-Nonsense Nutrition for Kids*. New York: Pocket Books, 1986.
Question-and-answer format arranged by age and age-related concerns, with sections on illness, dental health, and allergies by two registered dieticians and professors of nutrition. Available in hardcover and paperback.

Natow, Annette, Ph.D., R.D., and Jo-Ann Heslin, M.A., R.D. *The Pocket Encyclopedia of Nutrition*. New York: Pocket Books, 1986.
Dictionary of nutritional terms, with fuller coverage of particular topics. Includes appendix of nutritional analysis of foods. Paperback.

Prudden, Bonnie. *Fitness From Six to Twelve*. revised edition. New York: Ballantine, 1987.
Exercise regimes and introduction to a variety of sports. Paperback.

Prudden, Suzy. *Suzy Prudden's Exercise Program for Young Children*. New York: Workman, 1983.
Step-by-step exercise manual for parents and children (ages four weeks to four years), includes special section on baby massage. Paperback.

Satter, Ellyn, R.D., A.C.S.W. *How to Get Your Kids to Eat . . . But Not Too Much*. Bull, 1987.
The principles of nutrition and feeding from nipple through the teen years are presented by a dietician who is also a therapist. Specific advice and strategies are shared with insight, care, and

humor. Issues of concern to special needs children are also included. Paperback.

Sears, William, M.D. *Creative Parenting: How to Use the Attachment Parenting Concept to Raise Children Successfully from Birth Through Adolescence*. Revised and updated edition. New York: Dodd, Mead & Co., 1987.

Chapters in this overall guide focus on nutrition in pregnancy, breast- versus bottle-feeding, tips for breast-feeding, weaning, infant feeding, eating habits, and childhood obesity. Detailed, practical advice. Paperback.

Smith, Lendon, M.D. *Feed Your Kids Right: Dr. Smith's Program for Your Child's Total Health*. New York: McGraw-Hill, 1979.

The connections between diet, disease, and personality are explored. Levels of health and health profiles are established to help you understand the significance of fluctuations in your child's well-being. Available in hardcover and paperback.

Van Leuven, Nancy. *Food to Grow On (A Parents' Guide to Nutrition)*. Pownal, VT: Storey Communications, Inc., 1988.

A warm and lively book, filled with nutritional advice from pregnancy through those first school lunch boxes. Includes advice on table manners, party ideas, coping with junk food, eating out, and wholesome recipes.

Warner, Penny. *Healthy Snacks for Kids*. Concord, CA: Nitty Gritty, 1983.

Easy-to-prepare, tasty, and healthful recipes by child-development expert Penny Warner. Paperback.

Warner, Penny. *Super Snacks for Kids*. New York: St. Martin's, 1985.

More than 200 nutritious and creative treats, drinks, and meals. Easy to make, no added salt or sugar. Paperback.

The Womanly Art of Breastfeeding, 3d ed. Franklin, Park, IL: La Leche League, 1981. Reprint New York: New American Library, 1983.

Comprehensive, reassuring, detailed, and authoritative. Available in hardcover and paperback.

Nutrition—Juvenile Titles

Burns, Marilyn. *Good For Me!: All About Food in 32 Bites.* Illustrated by Sandy Clifford. Boston: Little, Brown (A Brown Paper School book), 1978.

Although no longer in print, this title alone will reward your visit to the library. It offers an engaging look at food and diet and provokes reflection on one's own eating habits. Informative fun for elementary-school-age children.

Carle, Eric. *The Very Hungry Caterpillar.* New York: Putnam, 1981.

This cleverly formatted and gloriously illustrated picture book tells the story of a little caterpillar who eats his way through the days of the week. His subsequent stomachache is relieved by munching a green leaf. The caterpillar eventually becomes a butterfly. For ages 2–6.

Cobb, Vicki. *Science Experiments You Can Eat.* Philadelphia: Lippincott, 1972.

Using the kitchen as a science laboratory. For elementary- and middle-school children.

Easy Menu Ethnic Cookbook (Series). Minneapolis: Lerner Publications.

An outstanding and attractive series featuring familiar and exotic cookery from such places as Vietnam, Norway, France, Italy, and Poland. Each title offers clear, authentic recipes, holiday treats, and a brief overview of foods and customs and is illustrated with mouth-watering photographs. For elementary-school children.

Ehlert, Lois. *Growing Vegetable Soup.* San Diego: Harcourt Brace Jovanovich, 1986.

From seed to cooking pot, follow the process of growing vegetable soup. The simple text is accompanied by intensely colored graphics and a recipe for this healthful dish. For ages 2–6.

George, Jean Craighead. *The Wild, Wild Cookbook—A Guide for Young Wild-Food Foragers.* Illustrated by Walter Kessell. New York: Crowell, 1982. Available in hardcover and paper.

A field guide for finding, harvesting, and cooking wild plants by the author of *My Side of the Mountain* and *Julie of the Wolves*. For elementary- and middle-school children with adult supervision.

Giblin, James Cross. *From Hand to Mouth: Or, How We Invented Knives, Forks, Spoons, and Chopsticks and the Table Manners to Go with Them.* New York: Crowell, 1987.
The title says it all. Filled with facts and humorous tidbits to give anyone's mealtime a conversational boost. A social history for elementary-school children and adults.

Greene, Karen. *Once Upon a Recipe: Delicious, Healthy Foods for Kids of All Ages.* New Hope, PA: New Hope Press, 1987.
More than fifty fast and easy recipes, with allusions to children's literature and cooking tips. Family fun. Paperback.

Isenberg, Barbara, and Marjorie Jaffe. *Albert the Running Bear's Exercise Book.* Illustrated by Diane de Groat. New York: Clarion Books, 1984.
Friend Violet teaches an out-of-shape Albert a wide variety of exercises, correct breathing, and safety rules. For ages 5–9. Available in hardcover and paperback.

Jones, Hettie. *How to Eat Your ABC's: A Book About Vitamins.* Illustrated by Judy Glasser. New York: Four Winds, 1976.
This clear and lively presentation of the role vitamins play in nutrition includes the importance of natural, unrefined foods, fun-to-solve "eating problems," and sample menus. For elementary-school-age children. Out of print.

Landau, Elaine. *Why Are They Starving Themselves?: Understanding Anorexia Nervosa and Bulimia.* New York: Messner, 1983.
Competent, nonsensational overview of two sister eating disorders. For adolescents.

Lukes, Bonnie L. *How to Be a Reasonably Thin Teenage Girl (Without Starving, Losing Your Friends or Running Away from Home).* New York: Atheneum, 1986.
Sound advice, reassurance, and support for a healthier lifestyle and better self-image. For adolescents and preadolescents.

Seixas, Judith S. *Junk Food—What It Is, What It Does.* Illustrated by Tom Huffman. New York: Greenwillow (Read-alone), 1984.
For beginning readers.

Showers, Paul. *What Happens to a Hamburger,* rev. ed. Illustrated by Anne Rockwell. New York: Crowell (A Let's-Read-and-Find-Out Science Book), 1985.
How our bodies make use of the good things we eat, told in clear and simple language with appealing illustrations. For ages 4–10.

Stein, Sara Bonnett. *The Kids' Kitchen Takeover.* New York: Workman, 1975.
More than 120 things to cook, make, and grow. Paperback.

Tornburg, Pat. *The Sesame Street Cookbook.* Illustrated by Robert Dennis. New York: Platt & Munk (a division of Grosset & Dunlap), 1978.
Simple and fun recipes for small children to prepare.

Weiner, Michael. *Bugs in the Peanut Butter: Dangers in Everyday Food.* Boston: Little, Brown, 1976.
This question-and-answer-format book delves into a variety of nutrition issues, including diet, health, additives, and inspection. Out of print.

What's to Eat? And Other Questions Kids Ask about Food. United States of Department of Agriculture Yearbook 1979.
Written for the International Year of the Child to bring the story of food and nutrition to children. Paperback.

Willey, Margaret. *The Bigger Book of Lydia.* New York: Harper & Row, 1983.
Lydia hates being small. Michelle is obsessed with becoming small and develops the symptoms of anorexia. The two girls share a special friendship, combining their strengths to overcome their problems. Insightful fiction for adolescents. A 1983 American Library Association Best Book for Young Adults. Paperback.

Index

••••••